Empowerment Through Reflection: The narratives of healthcare professionals

Other titles in the series:

- *Reflection: Principles and practice for healthcare professionals* by Tony Ghaye and Sue Lillyman
- *Effective Clinical Supervision: The role of reflection* edited by Tony Ghaye and Sue Lillyman
- *Caring Moments: The discourse of reflective practice* edited by Tony Ghaye and Sue Lillyman
- *The Reflective Mentor* by Tony Ghaye and Sue Lillyman

Empowerment Through Reflection: The narratives of healthcare professionals

edited by

Tony Ghaye, Dave Gillespie and Sue Lillyman

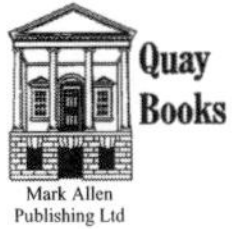

Quay Books Division, Mark Allen Publishing Group
Jesses Farm, Snow Hill, Dinton, Wiltshire, SP3 5HN

British Library Cataloguing-in-Publication Data
A catalogue record is available for this book

ISBN 1 85642 043 4

Printed in the UK by The Cromwell Press, Trowbridge, Wiltshire

Contents

Contributors

Tony Ghaye Cert Ed, BEd (Hons), MA (Ed) PhD
Professor of Education and Director of the Policy into Practice Research Centre, University College, Worcester

In my working life I have been fortunate in being able to work with and learn from a very wide range of professionals, including nurses, midwives, health visitors, GPs, social workers, police and probation officers, therapists of various kinds, osteopaths and school teachers. I have also experienced the privilege and challenge of working with individuals and communities in the Third World and in emerging nations in North Africa and the Middle East. All this experience has energised my commitment to inter-professional learning and multi-disciplinary working to help to improve what we do with and for others. I see reflective practice and action research as a central part of my work on quality of life issues. I have just completed the largest survey of its kind undertaken in the UK into young people's attitudes towards, and behaviours in relation to, illicit drugs and alcohol. This contributed to improvements in service policy and practice. I am the founder and editor-in-chief of the new multi-professional international Carfax journal, 'Reflective Practice'.

Dave Gillespie RMN, BSc (Hons)
Staff Nurse, Worcester

I am a registered mental nurse living and working in Worcester, England. After qualifying in 1993 I decided to continue my education at a higher level. I engaged in a BSc (Hons) degree course in Advanced Professional Studies for registered nurses at University College, Worcester. I gained a first class award and, subsequent to this, felt encouraged to pursue my studies further. I am currently a research graduate, again at University College, Worcester, working towards a PhD which focuses upon issues of power and empowerment in mental health nursing. In addition to my academic pursuits, I am an avid follower of hard rock and blues music, and I play the guitar badly. I play the drums a little better, having performed with groups in and around Worcester since 1981.

Sue Lillyman MA, BSc (Nursing), RGN, RM, DPSN, PGCE (FAHE)
Faculty Head of Quality Assurance, Faculty of Health and Community Care, University of Central England

Having qualified as a registered general nurse in 1980 and as a midwife in 1983, I worked in various areas, including intensive care, gynaecology and care of the elderly, and rehabilitation and acute medicine until entering nurse education in 1989. Having transferred with the Colleges of Nursing into the University of Central England, I worked as a senior lecturer within the Personal Development Unit for the Faculty of Health and Community Care and in 1997 took up my current role as Faculty Head of Quality Assurance. My teaching responsibilities have been with post-registration nurses undertaking diploma, degree and masters courses in nursing and collaborative community care for healthcare workers. Specialist areas of interest for me include care of the elderly, reflective practice, competence in practice, critical thinking and professional issues. I am soon to complete a PhD at University College, Worcester on the impact of reflection on nursing work.

Jan Quallington RN (GEN), ENB 249, Cert Ed (FE), BEd (Hons), MA
Senior Lecturer, University College, Worcester

My career in general nursing was spent largely in acute medicine and intensive care. During that time I learned to appreciate the need to value each individual patient and to approach their individual care as a unique challenge and privilege. These values have remained with me in my current role as a senior lecturer. My interest in nursing ethics was fostered by the successful completion of an MA in medical ethics. I am an enthusiastic advocate of the need to integrate practical ethics into everyday nursing practice.

Ian Stuart-Hamilton MA, PhD
Professor in Psychology, University College, Worcester

My research career has primarily been in gerontological research. After an initial period working jointly for the Institute of Psychiatry and Manchester University's Age Concern Centre on the intellectual effects of Alzheimer's disease, I co-authored an MRC-funded project to examine the effects of ageing on reading and spelling skills. Subsequent to this, I have written extensively about the effects of senescent ageing on the performance of traditional Piagetian and other 'childhood' tasks, educational gerontology and on changing images of ageing by both older and younger adults. I am editor/co-editor of two textbooks on ageing and am the sole author of five other textbooks, one of which, *The Psychology of Ageing* (Jessica Kingsley Publishers, 1994), is entering its third edition and has been translated into six languages.

Paul A Ward BA (Hons), DIP Nursing, RMN
Community Psychiatric Nurse, Herefordshire

Having served in the Royal Air Force medical trades, I entered work in the NHS in 1987 as a paramedic. I entered psychiatric nursing in 1996 after graduating from Manchester Metropolitan University and University College, Worcester. I currently work as a CPN in Herefordshire.

Acknowledgements

We are indebted to Hazel Alley and Sue Hampton from the Policy into Practice Research Centre at University College, Worcester for their help in preparing this manuscript and their enduring patience as we edited and then re-edited the text. We also owe an enormous debt of thanks to the many colleagues, students and patients who have inspired us to write this book. We hope that, in some way, this book might help us all to more richly understand our worlds.

The Editors
May, 1999

Introduction
Discussing the undiscussable

Tony Ghaye, Dave Gillespie and Sue Lillyman
May, 1999

This book is a challenging one aimed at individuals studying towards an academic qualification and having an understanding of reflection and reflective practice. You may feel uncomfortable when you read it as it discusses some very difficult issues in the management and delivery of healthcare. It touches upon some things that you may think and experience but cannot voice, or feel you can do much about. The book uses different languages: provocative, emotional, questioning, political but always, hopefully, professional.

The book aims to explore the links between empowerment and reflection. To do this we have had to examine notions of power and reality as they are known and experienced in a variety of healthcare contexts. The book is therefore divided into two parts.

Part 1 contains four reflective accounts which look at a variety of worlds of healthcare work and the struggles, hopes, frustrations and achievements of those portrayed. The book, therefore, begins with practice. In *Part 1* such issues as ethics, gender, age, voice, control, care, power, powerlessness, liberation, oppression, freedom and empowerment are brought into the open and allowed to breathe.

Part 2 reflects on the earlier portraits of practice. In doing so, it attempts to make more sense of practice, and 'positions' what has been told in relation to a more detailed discussion of conceptions of empowerment, power and reality. We argue that 'empowerment through reflection' might usefully be understood in relation to the important work of Paulo Friere, of Michel Foucault and of Jurgen Habermas.

We hope this book helps you to see your world more clearly — what serves to oppress, silence, liberate and empower. We hope you enjoy it.

Part I

The narratives of healthcare professionals

1

Ethical reflection: A role for ethics in nursing practice

Jan Quallington

Introduction

Ethics is increasingly seen as being fundamental to good nursing practice. All recent nursing curricula have an ethics theme and students of nursing are encouraged to study normative ethical theories in order to facilitate debates about the complex dilemmas inherent in healthcare. This is, of course, a necessary pursuit but ethics is not merely a cognitive activity restricted to the hypothetical; ethics has a very real contribution to make to practice. Ethics, like reflection, has at times earned itself the unjust reputation of navel gazing. Being a branch of philosophy it perhaps conjures up pictures of deep contemplation on the often insoluble questions of life. Professional ethics does inevitably have a contemplative component, however, its real purpose must be with the practical application to which this contemplation can be put. Ethics is only of value if it helps to inform and improve our practice. Professional caring is what nurses do. Caring has been described as 'the central and unifying domain for the body of knowledge and the practices of nursing' (Leininger, 1988).

Caring, because of its intimate involvement with others, is by its very nature an ethical enterprise. In order to care ethically it is necessary to reflect on the personal and professional values that we hold. These values directly influence our ethical reasoning, and consequently the actions that derive from that reasoning — both consciously and unconsciously. Ethical reflection, that is reflecting on practice using ethical frameworks to guide deliberation, should be a foundation stone for nursing practice. It is, perhaps, the key to excellence in practice.

It is my intention in this chapter to review how a group of nurses perceives and utilises ethics in practice; to illustrate through a small selection of nurses' stories a wider remit for nursing ethics which is both proactive and empowering.

Studies of nurses' perceptions of ethics and ethical decision making (De Wolf, 1989; Erlen and Frost, 1991 and Holly, 1993) indicate that ethics in nursing practice is frequently seen by nurses as a negative experience, invoking feelings of distress, frustration and disempowerment. If this profile of nurses' experiences of ethics is accurate, it is perhaps difficult to imagine that ethics can be used as a vehicle either to empower nurses or to enhance nursing practice. In the light of studies of the 1980s and early 1990s on ethical decision making in nurses (Gilligan, 1982; Gaul, 1987; Yarling and McElmurray, 1985 and Husted and Husted, 1991), I undertook a small qualitative study to review the current status of ethical decision making in nursing and how this affected the nurses' sense of personal control.

The study

In this study I interviewed a convenient sample of twenty general nurses, all working in an acute adult general ward environment in one district general hospital. All the participants were volunteers, were female and had each been qualified for a minimum of one year. Eight of the group had received some formal ethical instruction in their first level nurse education programme. The semi-structured interviews were conducted in the hospital informed by grounded theory (Glaser and Strauss, 1967). This approach was selected in order to prompt participants to relate actual ethical issues rather than to rely on responses to hypothetical situations which might not reflect the real issues that nurses encountered.

The interviews were structured around five main questions which had been identified by reviewing previous studies and by conducting a small pilot study of six participants.

1 What types of ethical decision had the participants taken part in in the previous two months?
2 How had they identified that these were ethical decisions?
3 What role had they played?
4 What strategies had they used to inform their decision making?
5 How satisfied were they?

The data were collected and analysed to identify common themes. Analysis of the interviews revealed several themes:

- ethical issues are the 'big' dilemmas of healthcare
- ethics is felt rather than thought
- opportunities to take an active role are restricted
- decision making relies heavily on intuition
- the structure in an acute care environment is disempowering.

Ethics are the big issues in care

When asked what ethical situations they had been involved with in the last two months, participants consistently related stories about the 'big' dilemmas of healthcare. One nurse talked about the discomfort she felt over the decision not to hydrate a patient who had had a dense stroke:

> *I knew he would probably die but somehow we didn't give him a chance. He was 74 — that's not particularly old these days. The policy is to wait and see if there is any likelihood of recovery before any active treatment is commenced in these cases, but how are you supposed to recover if nobody gives you any fluids or food? It's very hard trying to explain to the relatives why no treatment has been started. I don't feel the doctors understand what it's like having to make excuses about decisions that are nothing to do with you...*

Another nurse related this story:

> *We had a man in for an oesophagoscopy, unfortunately he suffered a ruptured oesophagus as a result of the investigation. He became very unwell and eventually ended up being ventilated. He was a Jehovah's Witness and his family made it clear that he should not receive a blood transfusion. This was respected, although it made his management much more difficult. The doctors did their best to try to persuade the family to change their mind. It was awful watching someone so ill when we had the power to help him.*

The issues that nurses chose to relate were all classic dilemmas; situations in which the agent is forced to select the least worst option. Nearly all of the issues cited revolved around questions of life and death. Questions about whether or not to resuscitate patients were cited by several nurses. None of the nurses in the study identified more everyday nursing activities as being ethical issues. A possible explanation for this apparent lack of recognition of ethics in day-to-day nursing practice, is that decisions of day-to-day care are often perceived by the competent practitioner as being unproblematic. It could be argued that these practitioners are demonstrating the skills of expert care as described by Benner (1984) — that is, actions and decisions being based on experience and intuition. However, it could not be determined from this study if this is the case. It could equally be argued from this evidence that nurses are not addressing the issues of ethics in everyday nursing practice. A great deal of nursing practice is still reliant on ritual, tradition and habit rather than on good ethical care initiated by an expert practitioner.

Ethics is felt rather than thought

It was evident through the interviews that ethical situations were recognised because of the feelings that they engendered; negative feelings of discomfort, anxiety and confusion:

> *You know something is an ethical incident because you feel uncomfortable about the way things are going, it preys on your mind... You just feel that something is wrong.*

Other nurses cited internal conflict and 'just not knowing what to do' as identifiers of ethical situations. This was in keeping with findings from De Wolf (1989) who listed the following factors as being the key identifiers of ethical issues:

- emotional reaction
- perceived time constraints
- personalising the situation
- communication failure
- disagreement about what constitutes right action.

Ethics, as it is perceived by these participants, is clearly a highly emotive issue.

Although feelings and intuitions are clearly very important influences, they are not always an accurate perception of things as they are in reality. They are likely to be influenced by our underlying personal and professional values, past experiences which may or may not be positive, and maybe by our own personal histories or prejudices. Consequently, it may be necessary to review these feelings using reflective techniques in order to attempt to validate them. Deconstructing the feelings and events — reviewing them objectively as if through the eyes of a stranger, may more accurately assist the individual to see the real issues. Application of ethical theories can be of great benefit to help the nurse to critically examine a variety of possible options. The added benefit of this is that it provides justifications for preferred choices. By decontextualising the issue it may be possible to identify more clearly what ought to be, and why. This is not to say, however, that all ethical questions can or should be solved by the application of pure rationalist arguments unencumbered by emotion. That would be to reduce the human state to that of the machine. Each situation will have its own individual context which needs to be added to the equation in order for the most appropriate solution to be found. Ethics is not an exact science and there are frequently several 'rights' and sometimes no 'rights' in any given situation. To make a decision without taking account of both rationalist and emotive perspectives would be to make an artificial and inappropriate decision. Clearly, a key feature must be to understand and be able to justify why a particular choice has been made.

Interestingly, *all* participants in this study identified feelings as being the predominant indicator of ethics, yet ethics is still largely taught as a dispassionate discipline. When the affective domain is clearly very dominant, this approach is obviously inadequate and is destined to leave the ethical agent feeling dissatisfied and with a sense that some vital component is missing. This certainly raises issues for how ethics is taught and what situations are focused upon.

What opportunities were there to take an active role?

Nurses in the study felt that their input into ethical decision making was restricted by the hierarchical structure that still exists in general hospitals. The nurses in the study felt that they were generally excluded from the process. Participants felt unable to contribute to ethical decision making and identified doctors as still taking the dominant role. These findings were similar to previous studies in this area (Yarling and McElmurray, 1985; Ketefian, 1989). This inevitably generated feelings of frustration and disempowerment and resulted in comments such as:

> *We are not consulted,... in fact I doubt whether ethics even comes into the equation, they just think they know best...*

None of the participants identified the patient as having a key role. Although this perspective was not pursued in the interviews it is not surprising, given the historical hierarchy that still persists in an acute hospital.

What strategies were used to make ethical decisions?

In spite of identifying that they did encounter ethical situations in their practice, none of the nurses articulated a consistent strategy that they used in order to attempt to resolve the issues they faced. Listening to the responses it was evident that the participants relied heavily on intuition; a gut response to ascertain the rightness or wrongness of a situation.

> *It is important to talk to your colleagues, but often you just know what is right because you know your patient.*

This response is representative of the feelings expressed by the other participants in the study.

None of the respondents interviewed made reference to the application of universal ethical principles and rationality. This could be due to a lack of knowledge of theoretical ethics, although eight of the sample had had some ethical teaching in their initial registration education. Gilligan (1982) argued that women make ethical decisions differently from men and would be unlikely to use normative ethical theories and principles as the basis for their decision making, relying much more heavily on those intuitive and emotive responses described by the participants in the study. All the respondents in this study were women. Kuhse *et al* (1993) has more recently argued that differences in decision making have more to do with occupation than gender and are partly a result of the education and training that influence the implementation of the process.

A second point that should be made in the light of the response quoted above is that it is often assumed by nurses that, as the professionals who spend the most time with the patients they are, therefore, the professionals who know them best. This may be true but may equally be an inaccurate perception. It is possible to be with someone for very long periods of time and never to get beyond the superficial; it is also possible to have a very short-lived but intense relationship with another individual. As a key member of the team, the nurse needs to be involved and probably has an extremely valuable contribution to make to ethical decisions, however, it is not necessarily on the basis of superior knowledge of the individual but rather on the basis of different knowledge. Most of us, even in quite extreme circumstances, show only those things about ourselves that we wish others to see. Presuming that we know what is best for others may be a dangerous road to tread. Yes, nurses have a contribution to make to big decisions but this is not an exclusive contribution. Collaboration between professionals, the patient and relevant others ought to be the preferred standard.

Active participation is inhibited

Participants identified the current hierarchical structure within acute care as inhibiting their involvement in ethical decision making. One nurse cited the need to be 'manipulative' in order to have her voice heard. Doctors' confidence in decision making may be a direct result of the style of education they receive which forces them into situations in which they have to make difficult decisions, and then take responsibility for those decisions. The experience of complex clinical decision making could lead one to suppose that doctors are better equipped to make ethical decisions than nurses, although this does not necessarily follow. Critical decision making is increasingly being featured in nursing curricula and it will be interesting to see how this impacts upon practice in the coming years. In addition, nurses need to be able to articulate their views more clearly to other professionals; no matter how right you are, it is not enough to say: 'I just feel this is right'. Justification for decisions is essential and is endorsed by the *Professional Code of Conduct* (UKCC, 1992).

Doctors, like other professionals, may feel unsure, isolated and lacking support when making decisions, and may welcome collaborative decision making. However, a study by Uden *et al* (1992) suggests that doctors are more likely to seek such support from superiors rather than requesting the cooperation of nurses. As one nurse cited:

> *I have frequently felt uncomfortable about treatment decisions that are made as to whether or not to continue feeding... they* [the doctors] *certainly don't invite opinions from others. When I have questioned them about their decisions, I've been surprised at how unsure they are about what to do.*

Rather than feeling excluded, nurses may need to promote the fact that they want to contribute. Surely it would be best in these extreme and difficult situations to work together and to value each other's contributions. The nurse may have a role as an advocate, or in providing alternative solutions. This in itself is empowering rather than frustrating and demoralising.

Whilst the results of this small study cannot be generalised, they nevertheless mirror findings in previous studies (Erlen and Frost, 1991; Holly, 1993). Ethics in nursing is still predominantly perceived to be restricted to the big dilemmas which, by their very nature, are — or should be — interdisciplinary. These issues invariably have no satisfactory solutions and leave those involved with feelings of frustration and dissatisfaction.

Having listened to nurses' stories over the years, I believe that there is a much wider remit for nursing ethics, and there is evidence that this is emerging. Nursing ethics is a discipline even now in its relative infancy, and the profession is still trying to establish just what nursing ethics is (Melia, 1986; Allmark, 1995). Although nurses failed to articulate day-to-day nursing activities as ethical issues, nearly all nursing practice has an ethical component. Ethics need not be something that is only ever brought out of a cupboard when all else has failed to find a satisfactory answer. Such an approach would inevitably engender negative feelings of frustration and disempowerment in the ethical agent. Indeed, in such cases there are often no really acceptable solutions to find. Instead, nurses can use ethics proactively; examining issues in everyday practice from an ethical perspective. Reflecting not only on what we do but also on what we ought to do. This process of ethical reflection should assist the practitioner to see that ethics is an essential component of all aspects of practice.

As a lecturer I have been privileged to hear nurses recount and explore values, experiences and dilemmas in practice. Perhaps these stories and others like them are the real issues for nursing ethics. The stories which follow are reproduced here with the kind permission of some practitioners. Student nurses are often well situated to identify the ethical issues in a placement area. They enter the environment without the hindrance of established practices and customs and often with a good measure of idealism and naïvety which allows them to question issues that others do not see or do not allow themselves to acknowledge. The first account is a story from a student on her first placement to a busy acute medical ward.

Story one

> *We have been caring for an elderly lady on our team. I don't fully understand what is wrong with her, but it's terminal — some kind of cancer, I think. She has developed pneumonia and her treatment has been stopped and she is just to have 'tender loving care'. Most of the time she is confused and doesn't know where she is. She has no close relatives and no one ever comes to visit her. She needs lots of nursing and I have been involved in doing her washes, mouth care and her observations. I always talk to her and explain to her when I have finished. Sometimes she doesn't seem to hear you, but when you go to leave, she clutches your hand. Even when she seems really confused, I think she is really scared. I try to stay with her as long as I can but there are so many other things to do. I think the other staff are beginning to avoid unnecessary contact with her because leaving her is so difficult and makes you feel so guilty. The trouble is this ward is so busy...*

This account is not included here as a criticism of the ward staff caring for this lady. They are, no doubt, under great pressure with many competing interests for their time. Rather, it is included as a reminder to constantly review those fundamental values underpinning practice, and as a reminder of the need to reflect closely on what we actually do rather than what we think we do in the light of those values. Ethical reflection in nursing enables the agent to identify what ought to be, and offers an opportunity to change practice in response to that reflection. Does this care really fulfil the unique role of the nurse (as identified by Henderson, 1966) to assist the patient to a peaceful and dignified death? Most of us would agree that it does not. In spite of the competing pressures, this lady should take priority over most other activities in the ward. She should have a nurse to sit with her, to support her and to assist her to a peaceful death. The justification, if one is needed, is both contextual and rational. Contextually, the patient is very clearly frightened and distressed, and it seems to be the *right* thing to do. More objectively and rationally, duty-based and consequence-based theories both agree that individuals are fundamentally equal, therefore we should be able to make an equal claim for care. Humans — simply because they are humans — are entitled to respect. If we are to be respected, our autonomous decisions ought to be listened to and, whenever possible, acted upon. Autonomy, where it does not infringe another's autonomy, ought to be respected (Beauchamp and Childress, 1994). In this case, the patient has clearly communicated her wishes to the nurses caring for her. There are, however, competing interests: obviously, time spent with this lady means that time cannot be spent with other patients. Other relevant important principles to bear in mind here are those of promoting good and doing no harm. The ethical decision is, therefore, who should receive priority? Ethical reflection may take the following form: whose interests should take priority and why? It could be argued that, with the exception of life-saving measures, the needs of the other patients could wait. Communicating this to those patients may be an important aspect of this issue. The dying lady's wishes have been clearly communicated and should take priority over other, less urgent wishes. This lady is dying relatively imminently; she will only die once; there is no room to get it right next time. The harm and distress that results from not being supported at this time is very real and cannot be rectified later. Washes, drinks, and even more complex nursing activities can be delayed. There is still a pervasive belief in nursing that getting the work done is the most important nursing action. Whilst this is undeniably important, the cost of achieving that goal should not be too high. If the ethical reflector combined the above reasoning with the knowledge that avoidance tactics are probably being used to protect the nurses from the discomfort engendered by delivering inadequate care, the agent would be obliged to review how this patient's care is being managed.

Ethical reflection requires that the nurse reviews the potential consequences of particular behaviours alongside fundamental values, whilst taking into account the particular context of the issue, in order to find a right way of acting.

Story two

> *We have lots of confused and demented patients on our ward. It seems that whatever you try to do for the best turns out wrong. These patients are frequently disruptive and interfere with other patients. It's not their fault; they don't know where they are half the time. The only thing that seems to work is if you sit with them. Obviously this has an effect on the other patients; just because they are sitting quietly doesn't mean they don't need any care. So what normally happens in the end is that the noisy and*

> *disruptive patients end up being mildly sedated so that they don't get so distressed. This doesn't really solve the problem, it just hides it.*

This is the voice of a frustrated and disillusioned nurse who feels that current strategies are inadequate but who is unable to offer any alternatives. The frustrations of feeling that one is not doing the job well and that the solutions one is using are not doing good and may even be perceived as harmful, may strike a chord with many practitioners. There are, of course, no quick fix-it solutions. This nurse has already taken the first steps towards improving practice. She has begun the process of ethical reflection. She has identified that this practice does not accord with her underlying values, and she has expressed the sense of discomfort that so often alerts us that this is an ethical issue. The next step is to begin to explore what the practice ought to be, taking into account the context and universal ethical principles. Reflecting on different options for achieving best practice might be the next step. This stage would preferably be done by the whole caring team, as it is likely to produce more diversity of ideas. It is important that any modifications in care management are agreed and accepted and consequently implemented by all those involved if change is to occur. Implementing and evaluating the most promising options enables the practitioner to regain a sense of empowerment and a control of their practice as well as potentially improving the patient's experience.

Story three

> *I work in a busy rehabilitation unit. The patients who we treat have usually suffered some catastrophic event which has changed their current and future lives. Patients are referred to us because they are likely to make significant progress and benefit from intensive rehabilitation. The staff in the unit are all committed to rehabilitation and promote a very positive attitude to the patients. Before they arrive with us, a rehabilitation programme is worked out with the multi-disciplinary team. We try to integrate the patients into the ward very early and encourage them to use the communal spaces when they are not booked for rehab. sessions. There is a fairly strict routine in the ward: the patients get up early so that they are ready for the physiotherapy and occupational therapy sessions at nine*

> *o'clock; lunch is served in the day room at half-past twelve and then there is a rest hour following lunch and prior to more rehabilitation sessions; the patients are usually tired at ten o'clock and the night staff try to get the ward lights out early.*
>
> *I was very proud of the positive environment that we convey in our ward until this was questioned by a patient who had been sent by their consultant to rehabilitate. No one had asked what they hoped to get out of the experience or indeed if they wanted to rehabilitate. They objected to getting up early in case the porter came to take them to the gym for their session. They had not eaten communally for some years and did not intend to start now. This caused me to stop and think about what we were doing, and for whom? Since that time the ward has begun to change; patients are much more closely involved in discussing what they hope to achieve and why they think they are with us. Appointment times are now made for all patients attending physiotherapy and occupational therapy, and are tailored to suit individual preferences where possible. Patients are asked where they would like to eat.*
>
> *These are only small changes and have interestingly met with some resistance from staff members, but this is only the beginning...*

This story needs little comment. It is a good example of a practitioner who reflected on their existing practice and who, whilst thinking it had been good, was prepared to review it. In fact, it resulted in her reviewing her own personal and professional values, and subsequently challenging the values of many of the team members. The result was an attempt to improve practice in the light of these reviewed values, the most prevalent of which has been the promotion and respect of patient autonomy. Listening to what the patients actually want, rather than what it is perceived that they want, has been a significant change in this unit.

It is easy to forget how powerful both the institution and we, the professionals, are. The needs and wishes of the individual patient can easily be overlooked in our attempt to impose norms and particular standards of behaviour on our environment. There is an old Chinese proverb that claims: what is ethically relevant is not understanding what it feels like to be me in that person's shoes, rather it is important to understand what it feels like to be that person in that person's shoes. This may be a very tall order, but it is an ideal to which we should be able to get closer if we reflect ethically upon our practice.

The three stories above are merely an illustration of how pervasive ethics is in nursing. The really important ethical decisions in nursing are those that occur in our everyday practice — the things that really make a difference for those in our care. It is about such things that we can pose the questions: 'How and why do I do the things that I do?' and 'What should I be doing?'

Ethical reflection affords us not only with the opportunity of 'extraordinarily re-experiencing the ordinary' (Schon, 1987, p.93), but also provides a vehicle through which we can find ways to change and improve the ordinary.

Ethics is a practical discipline, and ethical reflection is an essential tool for all practitioners. It need not be practised in splendid isolation but can be used as a team-building and strengthening tool. Exploring and implementing shared values and beliefs about care allows practitioners to manage change and to gain a sense of personal control in their work.

Nurses should, of course, contribute to the big ethical debates in healthcare, but there may be little satisfaction from such insoluble problems. More satisfying issues for nurses to grapple with may be those raised by ethical reflection:

- What are my values and philosophy of care?
- How well do I put my values and philosophies into practice?
- How flexible is my practice in accommodating individual needs?
- Do I encourage and support my patients to make autonomous choices for themselves?
- Can I justify and articulate the rationale and motives for my decisions, interventions and behaviours with reference to appropriate theory?
- Do I contribute effectively to the wider bioethical debate?
- How do I deal with the frustration and sense of disempowerment I sometimes experience in my practice?

Work by Bergum (1994) suggests that in order to care ethically it is necessary to refocus our professional foundations:

- to move away from a position of professional dominance in the relationship with those in our care and to move towards a position of true collaboration

- to adjust the view that only issues seen in the abstract can find the right answer and to move towards a position where the abstract is modified by the particular contextual issues
- to change the traditional focus of care from that of beneficence which is often paternalistic and controlling, to that of nurturance: the subtle change from 'caring for' to 'caring about'.

Ethical reflection can make a difference to patient care; it can also empower the nurse. By moving the focus of care to being more receptive to alternative ways of addressing issues and by working collaboratively with patients and colleagues, the nurse may be able to identify better ways of practising. There is unlikely to be just one right way of doing things; most decisions are a matter of judgement (Johns, 1998). Learning the language of ethics should assist nurses to deconstruct and reflect on practice; it will also assist in the articulation of that reflection which, in turn, affords practitioners the opportunity of justifying their practice and their decisions, both to others and to themselves.

It would be wrong to leave the reader with the impression that ethical reflection is easy or comfortable; often it is not. Practitioners may well share the sentiments of a nurse in an ethics class who was bemoaning the fact that I had made her role much harder:

> *Two or three times a day, now, I find myself really questioning my practice; at times it makes me feel quite insecure.*

Ethical reflection asks the practitioner to look for the ideal. I could be criticised for being unrealistic, but I make no apology for this idealism. If you aim for the ideal and, due to circumstances, settle for less, it must be better than settling for mediocrity or worse. In certain situations, ethical reflection may also enhance the practitioner's feelings of disempowerment. This is true when the issues that are being tackled are impossible to change. There will always be some things that we are unable to influence. If we have identified that this is indeed the case and that there are no creative solutions, we may need to let go until such time as the conditions have changed. Ethical reflection does not require practitioners to hit their heads against a brick wall. Knowing and accepting that some things are out of our control is an important lesson for us all to learn. Indeed, just knowing this may help us to cope with it.

I believe that ethical reflection provides practitioners with a platform from which they can gain a deeper understanding of their practice. I propose that it can improve practice and empower the practitioner, so leading to a greater sense of professional satisfaction.

Points for reflection

The following issues have been raised within this chapter:

1. In order to care ethically it is necessary to reflect on both personal and professional values.
2. Ethical reflection provides practitioners with a deeper understanding of their practice.
3. Ethical reflection can assist with empowering the nurse.
4. Utilisation of ethics is intrinsically linked with practice.

References

Allmark P (1995) Uncertainties in the teaching of ethics to students of nursing. *J Adv Nurs* **22**: 374–8

Beauchamp T, Childress J (1994) *Principles of biomedical ethics.* Oxford University Press, New York

Benner P (1984) *From Novice to Expert: Excellence and Power in Clinical Nursing Practice.* Addison-Wesley, California

Bergum V (1994) Knowledge for Ethical Care. *Nurs Ethics* **1** (2): 71–9

De Wolf M (1989) Ethical Decision Making. *Semin Oncol Nurs* **5**: 77–81

Erlen J, Frost B (1991) Nurses' perceptions of powerlessness in influencing ethical decisions. *West J Nurs Res* **13** (3): 397–407

Gaul A (1987) The effect of a course in nursing ethics on the relationship between ethical choice and action in baccalaureate nursing students. *J Nurs Educ* **26** (3): 113–7

Gilligan C (1982) *In a different voice: psychological theory amd women's development.* Harvard University Press, Cambridge

Glaser B, Strauss A (1967) *The discovery of grounded theory: Strategies for qualitative research.* Aldine Publishing Company, New York

Henderson V (1966) *The nature of nursing: a definition and its implications for nursing practice, research and education.* Macmillan, New York

Holly C (1993) The ethical quandaries of acute care nursing practice. *J Prof Nurs* **9** (2): 110–5

Husted G, Husted J (1991) *Ethical Decision Making in Nursing.* Mosby, St Louis

Johns C (1998) Unravelling the ethics of a good decision. *Nurs Crit Care* **3** (6): 281–2

Ketefian S (1989) Profession and bureaucratic role conceptions and moral behaviour among nurses. *Nurs Res* **34**: 248–53

Kuhse H, Singer P, Rickard M, *et al* (1993) partial and impartial ethical reasoning in health care professionals. *J Med Ethics* **23**: 226–32

Leininger M (1988) *Caring: An essential human need.* Wayne State University Press, Detroit

Melia K (1986) The task of nursing ethics. *J Med Ethics* **20**: 7–11

Schon DA (1987) *Educating the reflective practitioner.* Jossey Bass, London

Uden G, Norberg A, Lindseth M, *et al* (1992) Ethical reasoning in nurses' and physicians' stories about care episodes. *J Adv Nurs* **17**: 1028–34

UKCC (1992) *Professional Code of Conduct.* UKCC, London

Yarling, McElmurray (1985) The moral foundation of nursing. *Adv Nurs Sci* **8** (2): 63–73

Suggested reading

- *Nursing Ethics: An international journal for healthcare professionals.* Arnold Hodder Headline plc, London

2

Taking it on the chin

Paul Ward

Project 2000 RMN training, 19 August 1996

Final placement: acute psychiatric admission ward

Third shift: early

I was punched in the face by a patient today!

A new admission had come in overnight. A 32-year-old woman with a history of manic-depression who was currently hyper-manic. It had been a compulsory admission under Section 3 of the Mental Health Act (DoH, 1983), and this was the main source of her anger. The woman was extremely active, wandering the ward and regularly trying to leave. Her mode of speech was causing some problems, as she talked fast and furiously to anyone who would listen. In fact, it did not matter whether anyone was actually listening or not; she would shout at them anyway. Shout about the injustice of being 'imprisoned' there against her will. Shout at the nurses, using as many expletives as possible. She would be personally insulting and seemed to be particularly adept at targeting personal characteristics about which the individuals singled out were obviously sensitive. This was causing problems with other patients whose reactions were varied, depending on their current problems. For some the woman's behaviour fed into their paranoia; for others she was the devil come to torment them. One patient sat quietly brooding. He was always a powder keg waiting to blow and the general feeling was that this woman was likely to be the match to light the fuse. Other, more sensitive souls would scuttle away, sobbing — everything felt uneasy and unpredictable.

The situation was also causing problems for the caring team. The night staff were looking particularly jaded. They had been on the go since midnight and their patience was wearing thin. The sight of the day staff drifting in was obviously a blessed relief.

As a student nurse it seemed to go with the territory that I got all the jobs which the permanent staff disliked. I found it difficult to address this and to enter any meaningful discussion on the subject. 'We have all had to cope with crap as students. How else are you going to learn?' was the usual reply from other nurses. I was therefore assigned to 'closely observe' the woman. This is also known as 'one-to-one', 'level one' or 'level three' care, depending on where you work. It involves virtually shadowing the person, ensuring that they stay on the ward and that they come to no harm either from their own or others' actions. In theory this seems fairly straightforward — perhaps the only alternative to locked wards. In practice it is a complete nightmare, both for the observer and for the observed. It ensures that the nurse ends the shift feeling both drained and dehumanised from constant abuse. It is certain that the patient feels the same, but he or she cannot go home at the end of the session. Instead there is another fresh face to contend with. The procedure also appears to serve the function of making the patient's symptoms worse: increasing frustration, paranoia, and anger and then leading inevitably to aggression and violence directed towards the perceived oppressors.

This was my fate for the day, and my worst fears were realised. The more I followed the woman, the more she tried to lose me. The more I tried to communicate with her, the more she twisted my words and abused me. I felt inexperienced, and ill-equipped to deal with the situation. The other members of staff found my discomfort and embarrassment a great source of amusement. It was plainly obvious that the woman was finding the situation of a six feet four male following her around and watching her every move very threatening, as anybody would. Every effort on my part to communicate this perception to the qualified staff nurses seemed to fall on deaf ears. I felt that they were thinking I was trying to get out of the job — a job that was plainly the most difficult that day and needed an experienced approach to avoid a disaster occurring.

I was constantly assured that this was what psychiatric nursing was all about and that I would soon get used to it — this was the only way to learn. Perhaps this was true, but surely some guidance might be useful. As usual, my mentor was on a different shift and everyone said, 'Talk to her when you see her'. All well and good, but I needed it there and then — help!

It all came to a head when, after one particularly long tirade, the woman bolted up the ward towards the main door. I was in pursuit, trying to maintain any remaining shred of dignity that I thought either of us might have. As I rounded the corner, I came up against what felt like a brick wall but what was, in fact, a well-aimed fist to my jaw. I reeled back, mostly in surprise, tripped against a chair and fell flat on my back. Before I was able to gather my senses, male staff were everywhere.The woman was restrained using holds which, I am sure, have never appeared in any recognised control and restraint manual, and then marched to her room. The ward had suddenly become alive; other patients were ushered into the day room, keys jangled, syringes were drawn up and doors banged, whilst I nursed the mother of all headaches. Where had all these people been when I had needed them earlier? Nothing happened after that, except that I became the butt of the joke for the rest of the shift and I was asked to fill in a form about what had happened. That was it. The incident was soon forgotten. Not by myself, however. I had no physical scars but I was left feeling angry, humiliated and let down by my colleagues.

We, as mental health professionals, are generally perceived as all-powerful in the eyes of the patient (Johnson *et al*, 1997). This is by dint of our 'legitimate power' because our actions are sanctioned by society, and our 'expert power' because we are seen to have insight and skill (Price and Mullarkey, 1996). Generally, this professional power is accepted by most people under our care because they know they ultimately hold the trump card — they can refuse treatment and discharge themselves if necessary. This, however, was not so for my Sectioned patient — she could not leave or refuse treatment; I was her gaoler and tormentor, acting on behalf of an oppressive regime. The balance of power was tilted in my favour, yet why did I feel so disempowered? Maybe Price and Mullarkey (1996) have the answer:

> *... paradoxically, the client potentially holds the most powerful factor in the relationship: namely resistance, in particular to an authority figure — the nurse.*
>
> (p.17)

Certainly she resisted in the only way she knew how — by hitting back. It felt that this was her 'right' and there was nothing I could do about it. Maybe she knew that she could get away with it because, after all, that is what mentally ill people do, is it not? This seems to be the popular perception — that surely we cannot expect to work with the mentally ill and not get hit now and then? We must accept it, its all part of the job, an occupational hazard. Is this really how it is? Something that has always happened and will always happen? Is it something that we cannot change — psychiatric patients will be aggressive and violent, and psychiatric nurses the natural targets?

The important issue here seems to be that nurses feel disempowered when faced with aggressive and violent situations, and that perhaps the only way they can feel empowered in relation to this is to respond to like with like — they are human after all (Chambers, 1998). This response is perhaps legitimised by official control and restraint training. How can nurses empower themselves and move away from the 'accept it and respond when necessary' approach that appears to be the culture? I have a vested interest here to find an answer to this question because I do not want to continue with my chosen career as a sitting target, however inevitable the cultural norm expects that to be.

How should it be? I believe that we as psychiatric nurses (and I do include myself in this because I shall be fully fledged in two months — if this incident has not finally put me off!) should be exploring ways of preventing aggression and violence on the ward, thus empowering ourselves with prevention over cure and, in turn, inevitably empowering our clients so they do not have to use aggression and violence as a means of communication. In this way we would achieve a more even balance of power. Am I being naïve here? Will I, in a few years time, come to realise that this is simply how it is for psychiatric nurses and patients? Perhaps the stereotypical view that all psychiatric patients are violent goes much deeper than I realise, and manifests from a much wider social perspective. Certainly it is a view perpetuated by the media which influences the popular view, that anyone who works with psychiatric patients must surely expect to be assaulted at some point or another (Waterhouse, 1994). Psychiatric nurses and patients are, perhaps, as much influenced by the media as is anyone else.

There is a general perception that aggression and violence are problems which are increasing in society generally, and that it is understandable to expect such a trend to be mirrored in healthcare settings. Not only the output of the media, but also anecdotal evidence from the mental healthcare profession itself, continues to feed the expectation that aggression and violence is an occupational hazard. Breakwell (1989) acknowledges that values held by many in the caring professions show an acceptance of a certain level of 'tolerable aggression' from those in their care. She expresses the view, however, that these values may now be shifting towards zero tolerance, which I find encouraging in my current frame of mind.

When I performed an initial search through the academic literature on the subject, I was presented with many titles. Most have very recent dates and, at face value, seem to echo Breakwell's sentiments and highlight that I am not alone in being assaulted. The catalyst for the recent flurry of writing on the subject appears to have been a national survey conducted by the Health Services Advisory Committee (1987). Up until this point it seems that most research tended to be small, locality-specific and often anecdotal, making it difficult to generalise across the overall population of healthcare settings. Whilst the 1987 survey seems to have its own limitations, it certainly did much to highlight the experience of healthcare staff and to bring the subject on to the professional agenda. There is much evidence to suggest that nursing is a high-risk occupation for assault (Vanderslott, 1998; Stephen, 1998; Whittington, 1997) and the indications seem to be that the highest incidence of assaults to staff occur in psychiatric settings. Whittington (1997) reports that the number of assaults against nurses are skewed in these settings and quotes averages of one assault in every eleven days. Perhaps there is some truth in the stereotype?

Back in 1991, NUPE published a survey which found that 87 per cent of nurses interviewed were worried about violence. NUPE maintains that official statistics 'grossly underestimate' the level of violent threats made against nurses, with almost nine out of ten questioned saying that they had felt threatened at some time. All of these showed signs of distress lasting many weeks after the event (NUPE, 1991). It is also significant that Collins (1994) found a high rate of agreement with the statement:

> *Staff working with mentally ill people can expect to be physically assaulted some time during their career.*

Interestingly, one explanation given for this was that because there is so much literature suggesting that nurses can reasonably expect to be assaulted, it then becomes a self-fulfilling prophecy (Collins, 1994).

Some of the literature appears to support my own reactions to patient assault. Lanza *et al* (1991) reported reactions that included emotional, cognitive, social and biophysical responses, often lasting up to a year — well beyond the return to work. It was also found that staff often had to ignore or minimise their reactions in order to continue. This may explain the other nurses' reaction to my assault as it perhaps reminded them of their own experiences. It may also explain why I was the butt of their jokes and expected to join in. To laugh off and joke about assault is perhaps an understandable response when the culture persists with the perspective that this is part of the job description.

An interesting view offered by Janoff-Bollman and Frieze (cited in Murray and Snyder, 1991) perhaps helps to explain this.

They say that most people hold three basic assumptions which enable them to go about their lives and work in relative comfort:

1 A belief in personal invulnerability.
2 A perception that the world is meaningful and predictable.
3 A view of ourselves in a positive light.

These assumptions give a sense of safety, stability and self-esteem due to the perception that the world is an orderly place. The intense feelings that staff may experience when assaulted may be due to the breaking down of these assumptions. The person's world suddenly feels unsafe and unpredictable, there is a heightened sense of vulnerability, a feeling of being responsible for the incident and a negative self-image (for example, 'I am weak and foolish.').

This backs up both Lanza *et al*'s (1991) findings and my own experience that such incidents may be minimised, joked about, and any uncomfortable feelings laughed off as trivial by other staff. I would also agree with the view that the assaulted nurse can feel to blame for the incident and somehow be seen to have done something wrong. Such mechanisms serve to maintain a perception of control for those involved, whilst avoiding succumbing to their true feelings.

It is strange that we react in this way when there is no doubt that we all experience some form of negative reaction to violence and aggression. Poster and Ryan (1993) found that anger was the most reported emotional response immediately after an assault. Then, in the weeks following, other responses reported included anxiety, helplessness, irritability, sadness, feeling sorry for the patient, and feelings that the assaulted nurse could have done more to prevent the incident. This last was my own main feeling — surely there was more we could have done to prevent this happening.

It is encouraging that the literature highlights the effects which assault has on practitioners, but it makes depressing reading. There is a certain inevitability to it all that underlines one staff nurse's comment to me: 'You can't expect to become a psychiatric nurse and not get hit sometimes.' My answer to that is: 'Why the hell should I?' Why should we continue not only to feel powerless regarding patient violence and aggression, but also to sit back and just wait for it to happen? And why, when it does happen, can we react only in a knee-jerk fashion, using chemical or physical means to overpower the aggressor? Certainly, in this way we completely disempower our clients and ultimately perpetuate our own powerlessness. An endless cycle of disempowerment, each incident feeding the next.

If we could do as much as is possible to prevent violence occurring, surely this would go some way to breaking the cycle. But how preventable is violence? I cannot be the first to have asked these questions, so maybe I am naïve in thinking that it is possible. Thomas (1995), for example, has pointed out that no one has devised a satisfactory test to predict aggressive and violent behaviour and Allen (1997) concluded that risk assessment is an inexact science.

Logic rules out the notion that demographic variables, such as age, sex, race, education and socio-economic status, would enable the prediction of in-patient violence. Lanza *et al* (1996) concluded that sociodemographic factors were, indeed, unreliable as predictors and tend to be similar for the population in general.

I have noticed that psychiatric diagnosis is sometimes said to be a useful predictor, but this could present problems. Many patients can have more than one diagnosis, making it difficult to isolate the different effects. Also, it is apparent that two people with the same diagnosis do not necessarily behave in a similar way. Indeed, Davis (1991) concludes that:

> *patients with the same diagnosis may manifest different behaviour at different times, making diagnosis an unreliable predictor of incidents.*
>
> (p.590)

Despite this, a number of the staff nurses on our ward felt diagnosis to be a good predictor. One believed that: 'If you can stabilise the illness, then you stabilise the violence and aggression.' Another stated, 'You can pick out someone who's going to be aggressive by the type of illness that person has got.' The majority of staff, however, tended not to use diagnosis as a predictor alone but many did place significant emphasis on it. Whilst such diagnosis may be useful to 'put you on guard', it does continue to fuel the stereotype of violence in certain illnesses, such as schizophrenia.

Generally, stage of illness rather than diagnosis alone is a more useful predictor. Patients with psychotic disorders, for example, have greater potential for violence in the acute phase of their illness (Stuart and Sundeen, 1995). Sheriden *et al* (1990) noted that drugs and alcohol misuse play an important part in violent behaviour. Their findings suggest that substance misuse occurs more often in patients than is generally identified on admission. This is significant because I have since discovered that my assailant had in fact been misusing amphetamines for some time prior to her admission.

Sheriden *et al* (1990) and Blair (1991) view history of violence to be the most common factor associated with violence on admission. Palmstierna *et al* (1991) also found that people with a previous history of violence and drug misuse were significantly more likely to behave violently as in-patients. The authors conclude, however, that these findings have limited value for reliable prediction.

Davis (1991) reports on studies which highlight a variety of behavioural cues, which in turn correlate with violent behaviour. These include tension, mannerisms, posturing, suspiciousness and uncooperativeness. Whittington and Patterson (1996) found easily identifiable signs of imminent aggression, such as verbal abuse, abnormal activity and threatening posturing. Awareness of verbal and non-verbal behaviours such as these should allow the nurse to predict imminent assault and perhaps to take preventative action such as the employment of de-escalation techniques (Stevenson, 1991).

Psychiatric patients are likely to have low self-esteem and this can be exacerbated significantly by compulsory admission and enforced compliance with medication. As I have already observed, violence is, perhaps, the only way these patients feel they can achieve their desired needs.

Situational and environmental factors are believed to play a role in violent behaviour, and these include aspects of setting and the presence of staff and other patients. A number of writers have recognised that violence is interactive in that aspects of the in-patient's environment can affect that person's behaviour. Lanza *et al* (1994) maintain that situational factors are a key variable in the prediction of violence. They also cite other research which concludes that environmental factors have more significance than diagnosis in predicting violence.

A common occurrence in the studies is that violence is in some way provoked by environmental factors and is not simply the result of some underlying pathology. It is important to remember this.

Many of these factors are significant in relation to my own incident. Certain studies, for example, found that the number of incidents varied according to the time of day (Lanza *et al*, 1997). Eighty per cent of all incidents in Convey's study (1986) occurred between 8.00 am and 8.00 pm, and over a third were directly influenced by mealtimes. Lanza *et al*'s (1994) findings show that most assaults occurred in the ward corridors. Lanza *et al* also suggest that situations such as overcrowding, lack of space and privacy are important issues. Maybe it is noteworthy that my incident occurred in a corridor at around breakfast time. There is a significant amount of research to reflect upon in the field of aggressive incidents (Paxton *et al*, 1997; Pearson *et al*, 1986).

It is significant that many writers point to the environment as affecting the incidence of violence (Johnson *et al*, 1997). Our unit has narrow corridors with low ceilings and no natural light. The TV constantly blares out of the day room and smoke and music billow out of the smoking room next door — hardly conducive to relaxation and 'getting your head together'. Stevenson (1991) supports the view that a calm, quiet environment is essential in order to reduce anxiety and anger in patients experiencing frustration. Too quiet and calm, however, would surely induce boredom which is itself another factor influential in precipitating aggression (Stuart and Sundeen, 1995).

A report by Davies (1994) which investigated the conditions of a similar unit to the one where I work, indicates that one of the worst problems was that nurses could not see the patients due to the design and layout of the building. The layout of our unit, with its blind corners, has caused considerable problems — not least for myself, with a fist waiting for me as I rounded one of them.

More importantly for me, there has been significant interest in the issue of provocation. Blair (1991) maintains that provocation is an important risk predictor because the issues can be recognised, assessed and then appropriate interventions can be implemented to reduce the associated risks. He points to involuntary admission, physical or verbal limit-setting and staff attitudes as factors which can provoke a violent incident.

All of these factors are significant in relation to my incident. Certainly the fact that the woman had been admitted to our ward under the Mental Health Act was a key factor in initiating her violent response. This, together with limit setting in terms of preventing her from leaving the ward, added to the strength of her reaction. One staff nurse told me after the incident that, 'People who want to go out and are on a Section usually get aggressive.' Why was I not told this before? Going on this insight alone, my incident could have been predicted and thus prevented from reaching the stage which it did.

The use and effect of close observation appears a great deal in the literature, and most authors consider it to be a factor which provokes aggressive reactions. The ward policy states that if a patient is believed to be a danger to themselves or to others, then they must be closely observed.

Lowe (1992) cites the merits of monitoring the patient, yet most experienced staff believe that this often provokes aggressive and violent outbursts. The same staff nurse told me, 'Close observation causes or creates aggressive behaviour; people should always be aware of that.' This underlines the fact that *I* should not have been closely observing the patient — a staff member more skilled and experienced should have been given the task. Vanderslott (1998) cites studies which show student nurses to be the most likely grade of staff to be assaulted. Inexperience and poorly-developed patient relationships due to short-term placements, were put forward as likely explanations. Moreover, Lowe (1992) concludes that staff who are skilled in close observation will be able to recognise behaviour patterns, where ability places them in a very good position to prevent these patterns from escalating into violent action.

Morrison (1993) and Sheriden *et al* (1990) suggest that many violent patients view their staff victim as having provoked the attack. Davis (1991) points out that these patients claimed both provocation by staff and teasing by other patients as triggers for their violent behaviour. I am certainly aware that my following the female patient around may have provoked her attack on me. Ray and Subich (1998) suggest that staff attitudes can provoke aggression and violent behaviour. When staff act in an authoritarian, rigid or intolerant manner, patients may then try to regain control by using violent behaviour. Whittington and Wykes (1996) found that frustrating patients by limit setting, and intruding into their personal space stimulated them to respond violently.

Finally, Davis (1991) speculates that in-patient violence can be created by what he calls a 'norm of violence' on wards — there is an expectation that aggression and violence is acceptable and will be tolerated. This expectation may have evolved through an inflexible, non-therapeutic milieu which can make it difficult for staff to respond empathetically. The patients, in turn, see the ward as threatening and coercive, and perhaps believe that their only option is to react aggressively or violently. Such factors will create the very behaviour which staff are trying to control.

With some forethought regarding the possible effects of certain policies and procedures, many violent incidents could be avoided. And Rauter *et al* (1997) show that allowing practitioners to be creative within the limits of policy can reduce the perception of rigid, authoritarian staff.

Both aggressive and violent behaviour are complex concepts influenced by external and internal processes (Whittington and Wykes, 1996; Finnema *et al*, 1994). This makes accurate prediction a complicated task which is influenced by a variety of cognitive, perceptual and clinical skills (Morrison, 1993). Research examining the success of mental healthcare workers in predicting violent behaviour has found that their 'accuracy was significantly better than chance' (Thomas 1995), even when demographic factors were accounted for. Poster and Ryan (1989) point out that psychiatrists have made major efforts in recent years to stress that dangerousness cannot be accurately predicted. They found it interesting that, in spite of this, their study showed a high number of respondents indicating a belief that prediction is possible. A study by Fagan-Pryor *et al* (1994) concurred with these findings, and the authors cite other research papers which show a majority of nurses believing that prediction is possible.

A conclusion which could possibly be drawn from all this is that aggressive and violent behaviour is precipitated by a combination of factors. A few writers (Fox, 1998; Allen, 1997; Henderson and Robinson, 1997) have made some progress in developing risk assessment models. Significantly, these take into account multiple factors which can influence violent reactions.

So what does all this mean? Certainly I am now clear that prevention of violence is not as straightforward as I had hoped. Prediction is certainly multifaceted and can be highly speculative. However, we can go a long way in being aware of the danger signs.

The Royal College of Psychiatrists' guidelines on violence (1998) point to a number of factors which must be considered together. It is interesting that these do not seem to take into account the situational and environmental factors already discussed here, despite the importance which much of the literature places upon them. Whilst factors such as acute stage of illness, history of violence, drug and alcohol misuse, and so on, can go some way to putting staff on their guard, the guidelines still point to the 'respond if necessary' approach. All that seems to happen, for example, when an adverse risk assessment is made, is that more staff are drafted in which, in turn, serves the inevitable function of provoking a violent reaction. Around we go again!

An important point, which has become clear to me, is that we need to be more proactive when it comes to handling aggression and violence. This involves paying much closer attention to the role of situational and environmental factors in precipitating violent incidents. The literature appears to have been driving the point home for over a decade, yet it seems to have been largely ignored in the areas where I have worked.

Certainly, some environmental circumstances, such as the design of the building, are difficult to change but as new units are built, these factors must be taken into account (Davies, 1994). Other factors are possible to adjust, such as staff attitudes and how we present ourselves to the disturbed patient. Also, the practice of assigning the least experienced members of staff (that is, student nurses) to closely observe acutely ill patients should be avoided. As I move into becoming a fully-fledged staff nurse, I hope to be in a position to pay attention to these factors, or certainly at least to have the evidence on which to base my arguments.

As mental health nurses, we must be aware of the power relationship. In the eyes of the patient, staff members are all-powerful in terms of their professional power, yet the patient potentially holds the greater power through resistance (Price and Mullarkey, 1996). This is especially so where violent resistance is concerned. When faced with a violent situation, the natural human reaction is either to fight back or to run away. As psychiatric nurses we can do neither — our professional role will not allow it. The balance of power thus swings in the patient's favour until the nurse deems it necessary to use an officially-sanctioned means of 'fighting back', that is, control and restraint or medication. And so the struggle for power goes on until one side gives up. The one to capitulate is usually the patient, when either his or her symptoms become less acute or when he or she is medicated to the point of passive compliance, depending upon how cynical one's viewpoint is. This may seem an extreme view, and I may be bitter, but there is no doubt that this struggle for power goes on within psychiatric units up and down the country (Lipley, 1998). If, by paying some attention to the many factors highlighted in the literature and discussed here, just one violent incident a week is avoided and I never get hit again, then the time and effort will have been worthwhile.

In respect of my own experience and that of the profession in general with regard to aggression and violence, I am naturally taking the route that reflects on the issue from my own perspective. I am aware, however, that there is another and probably very different perspective — that of the patient. This leads us into the contemporary issue of service user empowerment. Certainly there are pertinent questions to be asked here, such as: What are the thoughts, feelings and experiences of patients with reference to aggressive incidents? Whilst not seeking to ignore the needs of service users or to minimise their experiences, I felt it important to focus on my own needs and those of my profession in developing a more informed practice. Of course, the needs and experiences of nurses and patients are both closely interlinked as well as standing in sharp contrast.

When patients become violent they are, perhaps, responding to their own powerlessness and, at the time of violence, briefly feel empowered. That is, they are gaining some control over external factors. Empowerment is generally expressed in this way and, argues Schafer (1996), is usually difficult to achieve. He asserts, however, that empowerment expressed in terms of control over oneself is more achievable. From this point of view we, as nurses, can create the conditions for this type of empowerment to grow, rather than trying to empower our clients *per se*:

> *Power comes from within. You can facilitate it, but you can't make it happen.*
>
> (Wallcraft, 1994, p.9)

With regard to violence and aggression, then, if we as nurses put into place the measures which help to prevent them, we create the conditions which empower our clients. Thus, we create a more positive cycle.

Initially I began this incident analysis with a view to redressing the power relationship between myself as a student and my qualified colleagues. I hoped to be able to fight my corner with the ultimate aim of avoiding being assaulted again. The analysis, however, led to my general perceptions that all psychiatric nurses felt disempowered when it came to patient violence, and that patient violence was accepted as an occupational hazard. It became clear to me that the only way I could hope to avoid being assaulted in the future was to look into approaches that would empower me and, hopefully, my profession. This seemed a tall order, but there are clearly numerous straightforward and well-researched measures which can be adopted. Many of these could be put into place with the minimum of fuss. Others may take more time but are still possible. I believe that, by implementing such measures, some headway can be made in redressing the balance of power, whether real or imagined, on acute psychiatric wards.

Points for reflection

The following issues have been raised within this chapter:

1. There is often a struggle for power within the clinical environment and there must be an awareness of the power relationship.
2. There is a need to empower the newly-qualified nurse to react professionally with the aggressive/violent patient.
3. The importance of reflection in understanding violence within the psychiatric ward, and its role in improving care.
4. Redressing the power relationship between the student and the qualified nurse.

References

Allen J (1997) Assessing and managing risk of violence in the mentally disordered. *J Psychiatr Mental Health Nurs* **4**: 369–78

Blair DT (1991) Assaultative behaviour: does provocation begin in the front office? *J Psychosoc Nurs* **29** (5): 21–6

Breakwell GM (1989) *Facing Physical Violence.* Routledge, London

Chambers N (1998) We have to put up with it don't we? The experience of being the registered nurse on duty, managing a violent incident involving an elderly patient: a phenomenological study. *J Adv Nurs* **27** (2): 429–36

Collins J (1994) Nurses' attitudes towards aggressive behaviour, following attendance at 'The prevention and management of aggressive behaviour programme'. *J Adv Nurs* **20**: 117–31

Convey J (1986) A record of violence. *Nurs Times* 12 Nov: 36–8

Davis S (1991) Violence by psychiatric inpatients: A review. *Hosp Community Psychiatry* **42** (6): 585–90

Davies F (1994) Killer Building Syndrome. *Guardian* 28 May: 6–10

Department of Health (1983) *Mental Health Act.* HMSO, London

Fagan-Pryor EC, Femea P, Haber LC (1994) Congruence between aggressive behaviour and type of intervention as rated by nursing personnel. *Issues Mental Health Nurs* **152**: 187–99

Finnema EJ, Dassen T, Halfens R (1994) Aggression in psychiatry: a qualitative study focusing on the characterisation and perception of patient aggression by nurses working on psychiatric wards. *J Adv Nurs* **19**: 1088–95

Fox G (1998) Risk assessment: a systematic approach to violence. *Nurs Stand* **12** (32): 44–7

Health Services Advisory Committee (1987) *Violence to Staff in the Health Services*. London, HMSO

Henderson S, Robinson D (1997) Developing a behavioural status index to assess patient dangerousness. *Mental Health Care* **1** (4): 130–2

Johnson B, Martin M, Guha M, *et al* (1997) The experience of thought-disordered individuals preceding an aggressive incident. *J Psychiatr Mental Health Nurs* **4** (3): 213–20

Lanza ML, Kayne HL, Gulliford D, *et al* (1997) Staffing of inpatient units and assault by patients. *J Am Psychiatr Nurses Assoc* **3** (2): 42–8

Lanza ML, Kayne HL, Pattison I, *et al* (1996) The relationship of behavioural cues to assaultive behaviour. *Clin Nurs Res* **5** (1): 6–27

Lanza ML, Kayne HL, Hicks C (1994) Environmental characteristics related to patient assault. *Issues Mental Health Nurs* **15**: 319–35

Lanza ML, Kayne HL, Hicks C (1991) Nursing staff characteristics related to patient assault. *Issues Mental Health Nurs* **12**: 235–65

Lipley N (1998) Trusts to get targets for reducing violence. *Nurs Stand* **12** (41): 8

Lowe T (1992) Characteristics of effective nursing interventions in the management of challenging behaviours. *J Adv Nurs* **17:** 1226–32

Morrison EF (1993) A comparison of perceptions of aggression and violence by psychiatric nurses. *Int J Nurs Studies* **30** (3): 261–8

Murray MG, Snyder JC (1991) When staff are assaulted. *J Psycholog Nurs* **29** (7): 24–9

NUPE (1991) *Violence in the Health Service*. NUPE, London

Palmstierna T, Huitfeldt B, Wistedt B (1991) The relationship of crowding and aggressive behaviour on a psychiatric intensive care unit. *Hosp Community Psychiatry* **42** (12): 368–75

Paxton R, Anslow P, Milne D, *et al* (1997) Evaluation of a new record system for aggressive incidents in mental health services. *J Mental Health* **6** (2): 149–67

Pearson M, Wilmot E, Padi M (1986) A study of violent behaviour among inpatients in a psychiatric hospital. *Br J Psychiatry* **149**: 232–5

Poster EC, Ryan JA (1989) Nurses' attitudes toward physical assaults by patients. *Arch Psychiatr Nurs* **3** (6): 315–22

Poster EC, Ryan JA (1993) 'At risk of assault. *Nurs Times* **89** (23): 30–2

Price V, Mullarkey K (1996) Use and misuse of power in the psycho-therapeutic relationship. *Mental Health Nurs* **16** (1): 16–7

Ray CL, Subich LM (1998) Staff assaults and injuries in a psychiatric hospital as a function of three attitudinal variables. *Issues in Mental Health Nurs* **19** (3) 277–89

Rauter UK, de Nesnera A, Grandfield S (1997) Up in smoke? Linking patient assaults to a psychiatric hospital's smoking ban. *J Psychosoc Nurs* **35** (6): 45–6

Royal College of Psychiatrists (1998) *Management of Imminent Violence.* RCP, London

Schafer T (1996) Empowering service users: the myth, the reality and the hope. *J Psychiatr Mental Health Nurs* **3**: 391–4

Sheriden M, Henrion R, Robinson L, *et al* (1990) Precipitants of Violence in a Psychiatric Inpatient Setting. *Hosp Community Psychiatry* **41** (7): 776–80

Stephen H (1998) Horrifying catalogue of attacks on nurses. *Nurs Stand* **12** (50): 9

Stevenson S (1991) Heading off violence with verbal de-escalation. *J Psychosoc Nurs* **29** (9): 6–10

Stuart GW, Sundeen SJ (1995) *Principles and Practice of Psychiatric Nursing.* Mosby, Missouri

Thomas B (1995) Risky Business. *Nurs Times* **91** (7): 52–4

Vanderslott J (1998) A study of incidents of violence towards staff by patients in an NHS Trust hospital. *J Psychiatr Mental Health Nurs* **5** (4): 291–8

Wallcraft J (1994) Empowering empowerment: professionals and self-advocacy projects. *Mental Health Nurs* **14** (2): 6–9

Waterhouse R (1994) Why did Georgina Robinson die? *Independent* 5 Dec: 17

Whittington R (1997) Violence to nurses: prevalence and risk factors. *Nurs Stand* **12** (5): 49–56

Whittington R, Patterson P (1996) Verbal and non-verbal behaviour immediately prior to aggression by mentally disordered people: enhancing the assessment of risk. *J Psychiatr Mental Health Nurs* **3** (1): 47–54

Whittington R, Wykes P (1996) Aversive stimulation by staff and violence by in-patients. *Br J Clin Psychol* **35**: 11–20

3

A nurse's career: Reflections from behind the learning curve

Dave Gillespie

All sorts of things happen to nurses; some good, some bad. The good things can take a variety of forms: seeing a patient who has been seriously ill getting better and going home, being involved in a supportive team who can be relied upon, having a laugh with colleagues from time to time. The bad things can include seeing patients becoming more and more poorly, potentially to the extent that they die; feeling unsupported by colleagues; feeling overworked and tired out, but still having to work. Nursing is an emotional roller coaster; the whole range of emotions is experienced. It can be extremely hard physical work, particularly in some areas such as care of the elderly. It may require tremendous watchfulness, for example on intensive therapy wards of which there is a variety. Nurses often work shifts which is physically very tiring. Add this to the emotional strain, and the problems nurses face begin to take shape. Those nurses working in the community require a responsible approach to maintaining an often very large case-load of patients. In their work, nurses can even be exposed to danger to themselves. Those working in accident and emergency, and in psychiatry would perhaps be most at risk from aggressive patient behaviour, although I have heard tales of violence occurring even on care of the elderly wards. So here we have an enormously difficult job; the sort of job where those doing it are certainly in need of some form of support.

The kind of support required may take a variety of forms: nurses may need help and encouragement from their immediate colleagues — the nurses with whom they work; they may need support from the medical staff they spend time with; and it should certainly be provided by those who manage nurses. Brewer and Lok (1995) identify the support strategies which management should be using. Often, of course, day-to-day experience is very different. Nurses, or any other group working closely together, can find themselves falling out with each other; working with nurses they particularly dislike being with — people who 'get on their nerves' and drive them mad. Many of the 'ideal' books about nursing would describe ways around this; how the problem can be avoided; how it is that all nurses can work happily together. In reality, this may prove very difficult. As far as the doctors are concerned, they may be a further source of discomfort to nurses, ordering them around and telling them what to do. And managers? Well, managers have their own targets to meet, their own goals to achieve, and these may often override consideration of their nursing staff. Nursing presence in management has diminished since the Griffiths report (Gabe *et al*, 1991) and, as a result, nurses' interests are now, perhaps, given less weight and attention. The working environment for the nurse can therefore be extremely difficult, and I have hardly mentioned the problems which patients can create.

I am a psychiatric nurse. I was registered in 1993, so to some degree I am a relatively 'modern' nurse as opposed to those who have worked in the 'profession' for many years. My training began in 1990. When I showed up on my first day, I was so anxious that I could hardly breathe. I was a member of a joint introductory group consisting of eight RMN trainees and twenty RGNs. We spent the first couple of months together before each going into our respective disciplines. The RMN group consisted of a most disparate bunch of people. I remember them all very well — different ages, sexes, backgrounds, classes and attitudes. But we got on well, and we needed to. We would be spending the next three years together.

My training was divided into a series of placements with various mental health services, interspersed with time in the classroom learning the 'theory of nursing'. The theory, I guess, was designed to turn us into 'ideal' nurses. However, it was often so divorced from reality that it was more or less meaningless. Not surprisingly, despite my early hopes and idealism, this disparity between theory and reality was to become a major source of tension throughout my nursing career. Despite my enthusiasm for all the theory thrown at me, I discovered that very little of it was applicable in the real world of psychiatric nursing. The theory-practice gap in nursing is well recognised (Conway, 1994). This is not to suggest that I did not enjoy my practical placements — I did — but it became tedious learning about the merits of talking therapies, of nursing models, of ethical principles and values, when apparently none of these things actually existed in practice and, when raised, were often resisted by already practising nurses. No matter how enthusiastic I or any of my fellow trainees might be about the theory, the die had already been cast; the attitudes of qualified staff were already set. Disillusionment was rife. The educators would try to paint a glossy picture but the cracks in the canvas were all too apparent: a lot of very fed up and burnt out nurses persisting in a job that simply made them feel more fed up as time went by. Still, as I rarely stayed in any particular place for more than a few months, there was always something new to look forward to and there was always the challenge of another theoretical assignment to meet, however unrealistic or impracticable it might be.

I remember my first year. I did placements in community, rehabilitation and — my biggest dread — on the general wards. Community was great. Lots of variety, a great mentor — one of the few who still had real enthusiasm for the job despite its pitfalls — and my first injections! On the first occasion, I shook so much that I could hardly hold the syringe, never mind actually stick it into someone. My head was full of doubts. I hated the idea of inflicting pain on someone, no matter how willing they might be. But I had no choice. I had to learn it; it was part of the job — a big part. Rehabilitation, or 'rehab' as it is abbreviated, was twelve weeks of what seemed interminable boredom. A very difficult job causing emotional problems for staff. This was also where I began to learn about the sad reality of psychiatry. I worked in a community home which aimed to rehabilitate people who had proved extremely difficult to help. People who had been 'dumped'. Most of them had been in hospital for decades and on anti-psychotic drugs for many years, and it showed. They were like the living dead, and 'they' thought they could rehabilitate these people. What were they thinking? In reality, it was all a charade — an attempt to achieve the unachievable. Everybody knew it was impossible, but every day the nurses would turn up to maintain this charade, moaning endlessly about the futility of it all. At least it paid the mortgage. This was not good. This was sheer pointlessness. There was no achievable goal; no salvation for these people. I hated every second of it.

The general wards were anathema to me. Highly structured, disciplined, procedural, dogmatic. Laden with apparently pointless ritual and highly hierarchical. Everyone knew his or her place and role — and the trainee psychiatric nurse was very much at the bottom of the heap. In class at college the lecturers would talk about moving away from task-oriented care, but on the wards tasks were the order of the day. Bed-making, washing, dressing, feeding, drug rounds, doctors' rounds, more bed-making, more feeding, more washing, changing. Remorseless, round and round in circles hour after hour, day after day. How ritualistic nursing can be (Walsh and Ford, 1989)! Patients came, and went — either home or to the mortuary, but there were always more to replace them; more to feed, wash, change, and so on. I think you get the picture. And where was all the theory? I could not see it. And the ward sisters? They were somewhat megalomaniac. And the staff nurses? Aspiring megalomaniacs? Perhaps there are fundamentally two types of people who are attracted to nursing: those who genuinely care and want to care, and those who like power. Those who care become trapped in the hierarchy; those who are into power get into power and make sure that those who care stay trapped in the hierarchy. A personal view, of course, but one I am sure a lot of nurses would recognise.

I then entered the dark world of acute psychiatry for the first time. My initial encounter with an acutely ill patient resulted in his asking me if I would like to fight him. I will never forget the glazed expression in his eyes, his emotionless face. The only response I could think of was, 'No, thanks!' So, maybe all the stories I had heard — about all the violence in acute psychiatry — were actually true, despite the reassurances to the contrary that we had been given prior to placement. Indeed, I encountered quite a lot of violence on that placement. Aggressive patient behaviour is fairly common (Warner, 1992). A staff nurse was seriously assaulted. He was attacked by a patient and had five teeth dislodged. Was this really what I wanted to do? At this time I had serious doubts. The ward itself seemed to be in utter chaos most of the time. There was very little of the tranquil environment I had envisaged. It was, for the most part, total bedlam. Some very ill people and some very stressed nurses. It was here that I witnessed, at first hand, some of the patient abuse associated with psychiatry. A male nurse hip-threw a female patient to the floor. Certainly, this patient was extremely taxing, but it was excessive to say the least. I also saw the effects of anti-psychotic drugs for the first time. Patients walking around like zombies, quite unable to sit still, pacing round and round the ward endlessly. I saw their bizarre behaviour. One wore towels around his head in a futile effort to block out the voices which were taunting him. Very sad. He was overwhelmingly tormented and seemed beyond help, despite the huge quantity of medication he was on. Nursing care appeared haphazard and disorganised. There was much disharmony in the nursing team — colleagues criticising each other, running each other down. It was a pretty sad state of affairs, all in all.

Well, that placement came and went, and then we were back in college again, being taught more theory which bore little relation to our experiences in the real world. We student nurses talked a lot about how things could be so much better; about how, when we qualified, things would be different; how we would change things. On reflection, we were a little naïve, but at least we were still hopeful and optimistic. More placements followed in psychogeriatrics, in the community and on substance misuse. I was, by now, in my third year of training and was due to qualify very soon. This was a nervous time. I felt under prepared, inadequate and racked with self-doubt. I would soon be expected to perform as a competent nurse. Also, I would soon be shouldering a great deal of responsibility. Was I ready? Was I hell! Sure, I had done the theory, but felt that my practice was well short of the mark. In fact, the last few months of training was where I really learnt. I had to take charge of the ward — what they called 'management' training. I had to make decisions, at least tentatively. And I had my 'finals' to sit. Anyway, it all worked out all right and, in August 1993, I qualified as an RMN.

I applied for one job and got it. I finished my training on the Friday — an emotional occasion for all the students in my group — and started as a staff nurse on the following Monday. My first day came as a rude awakening. I arrived on the ward to find that the other qualified nurse due to work that day had gone off sick. This left me in charge of the ward (which was in utter chaos), working with one nursing assistant. I was petrified. I contacted the person in charge of the hospital site and requested backup, which thankfully I got. Not a great start.

Anyway, I persisted and, as the weeks and months went by, things got better. I realised fairly early on that my training had only been the start of my education as a nurse. You don't really start to learn about nursing until you become a staff nurse. It is really practice that teaches you. A lot of what you come to know about nursing is borne out of experience, rather than the textbook. In actual fact, theory appears to be positively frowned upon by the majority of qualified staff. In my early days as an RMN, I maintained my enthusiasm for theoretical nursing in spite of the opposition of the other nurses I worked with. I think they saw me as something of a 'smart-ass' who would soon learn that nurses like me just do not succeed. There were so many things I did not like on the ward. The way, for example, that some nurses spent most of their time sitting in the office, chatting to each other rather than being out on the ward talking to patients. I became increasingly frustrated at the lack of time available in which to use any of the skills I had learned as a student. My job revolved around coordinating the nursing team, managing the ward, attending meetings, talking to other health workers and talking to the relatives of patients. Very little time was spent working with patients. Porter (1993) sees this as the needs of the institution coming before the needs of the patient. At this time I realised that I had a choice to make: because of the time constraints, I could either become a 'management-style' nurse or a 'therapeutic' nurse. I could not do both. Still full of the idealism instilled in me by my training, I decided to attempt the latter and devoted much of my time to my patients, admittedly to the detriment of my other duties. I was soon to come in for some heavy criticism from my seniors for this decision. I spent too much time with patients and not enough time tending to the running of the ward, maintaining ward order and the ward routine. I neglected my paperwork. I was gradually learning the things that were considered most important — and it seemed that patient care was not one of them.

So, at this time I was going through something of a 'nursing style crisis'. I was attempting to follow a rather ideal way of nursing in an environment where 'control' was the key issue. Control of patients — in this instance, psychiatric patients — was what seniors wanted. There are obvious reasons for this. Psychiatric patients who are out of control are not exactly safe. Those suffering from illnesses with symptoms potentially causing them to be out of control, in addition to being in an 'out of control' environment can easily become violent. I have seen it time and time again. Those suffering from suicidal symptoms need to have a close eye kept on them. If they don't, they may kill themselves. So, it was all about control of the ward; there was no space for 'therapeutic interaction'. There were not enough nurses to facilitate both. Control was the 'top dog'. This was, indeed, the reality which I faced at a time when the educational establishments were producing nurses who were highly therapy oriented. Hence the dilemma: do what you were trained to, or do what already happens — fit in, comply. Those nurses who chose not to comply would not be popular, as I found out. The nursing team on our ward had recently had a new ward manager who was trying to implement change. He was attempting to bring in new ways of operating, but was often met with resistance both from senior management and the staff already working on the ward. However, as time went by he did manage to implement some of his desired changes. They were basically good ideas but the problem they created for the nursing staff was that they were very demanding, requiring much more of them than they were used to. Anyhow, it all took place and this was all going on while I was a newly-qualified nurse, still wet behind the ears.

At this time, there seemed to me to be something of a divide within the team. Again it was related to the issues of 'nursing' or 'controlling' patients. Some nurses were interested in the former while others were attracted to the latter. The ward manager was more interested in control. He had to present a controlled ward to senior management; it would not have done his credibility much good to present anything else. He implemented a strategy to influence all nurses to prefer to control the ward rather than spending time with the patients. I suppose you cannot blame him. Failure in maintaining order can get a nurse into trouble (Porter, 1993). For those nurses who had been taught to place emphasis on therapy, this was an extremely difficult situation. Such nurses were generally the type who were not terribly good at being controlling anyhow. They were the sort who would attempt to make patients' lives a little easier, who would listen to their problems and have sympathy with them. This involved spending time with the patients, even possibly allowing the ward to become a little chaotic. This obviously created problems for the manager; his ward was perhaps not as ordered or as organised as it should be. Spending time with patients and having genuine concern for them, also means the willingness to protect them. Psychiatry has something of a dubious history. It has not always treated its patients too kindly. In fact, many psychiatric patients in the past were exposed to little else but abuse from staff. This is something which the discipline is currently attempting to rectify. Much abuse of patients has, in my view, been borne out of a number of issues. Psychiatric patients are difficult to nurse; they are often uncooperative, hostile, demanding, rude. The nurses who work with them are exposed to a great deal of problem behaviour which makes their practice very difficult. When faced with these kinds of behaviours, in addition to the other pressures to which nurses are exposed, nurses may react in an inappropriate fashion and the patient may come in for some hostility. I remember an incident which illustrates exactly this.

The following experience is one which has had a major impact on my nursing career in general. Reflecting upon it has caused me to reappraise everything. Thankfully, it occurred early in my time as a qualified nurse and it has led to my total reconsideration of nursing and healthcare provision. It was an early shift. I was making the early-morning drug round with a senior nurse who had many years' experience. There was a schizophrenic patient who was acutely psychotic. He was on a huge dose of chlorpromazine, a heavily sedative drug. The senior nurse asked me to call this patient to come and get his medication, which I did. After a few minutes he hadn't come and I was asked to call him once more. Again he did not come. At this point, the senior nurse seemed to 'lose her cool' completely and said that she was going to inject the patient forcibly. He had been detained under Section 3 of the Mental Health Act (DOH, 1983). I felt this was way over the top. Would it not be easier just to take his oral medication to him? It would certainly avoid any risk of injury to staff or patients. This particular patient had a history of violent behaviour. I had a decision to make. Did I carry out the senior nurse's instructions, or voice my concerns? Well, I chose the latter. I told the senior nurse that I did not agree with her decision. She marched me into the ward office and began to lecture me on loyalty and the importance of nurses sticking together. She was furious, almost out of control. I stuck to my guns and refused to agree with her. Eventually she gave up and said, 'Oh, do what you like then.' I went over to the patient and asked him to come to the clinic with me to take his medication orally, which he did — no problem. The senior nurse did not speak to me for the rest of the day; I had challenged her authority and she did not like it. But this was an ethical and professional issue. Why put staff and patients at risk when it could be avoided relatively easily? I could not understand where she was coming from. Was she seriously acting in the best interests of her patients? I did not think so. I thought she was creating a potentially dangerous situation and I could not collude with that. She was actually trying to demonstrate to the patient — in no uncertain terms — who was in charge, who was in control. I still remember this incident because it taught me so much about what nursing, perhaps only psychiatric nursing, is really about. It's supposed to be about caring, about empathy, about human concern, about helping. The senior nurse was wrong in so many ways. In my opinion, if we had done what she had suggested, then she (and certainly I) would both clearly have been breaking our Professional Code of Conduct (UKCC, 1992) — possibly clauses 1, 5, 9, 13 and 14. We would not have been upholding the spirit of the code in any way. That is why I acted as I did, because I felt that what was being suggested was completely unprofessional. It was also immoral and unethical. For the next year or so my life was made a misery by this nurse; she made it hell. But I am pleased about — no proud of — what I did. What the incident has caused me to do since is to think very seriously about the nature of nursing. I had originally been taught that nursing was about caring; about having concern and sympathy with the predicaments of those who are unwell, and doing what we can to help them. Simply that. However, my experience showed me that there is much more to it than that. Sometimes, it seems to me — though this may not be the experience of all nurses — that nursing is more about power than about caring. Indeed, for me in lots of different ways what it is *really* about at the end of the day, is power.

The issue of power occurs everywhere (Cheek and Rudge, 1993). It manifests itself in many different ways. I had experienced it as a student on the general wards, where the ward sister was revered and held in awe by her staff. On the psychiatric wards there is the ritual tea-making which is used to emphasise to the student their position in the hierarchy — rather like the tea-boy in the office. Nurses who have far longer experience than my own tell me stories about how, during his ward rounds, one consultant liked to have all the patients standing to attention at the foot of their beds waiting for his inspection, and with their beds perfectly made. In my own experience, I recall a consultant who would interview patients from the lofty position of his power chair on which he would swing around, staring up at the ceiling whilst lecturing them about the iniquities of their bizarre behaviour and what he was going to do about it. I remember the registrar who refused to take an alcoholic patient off a Section of the Mental Health Act because she thought he would drink again (this decision was certainly unethical and almost certainly illegal). There are also the managers who work on the other side of the hospital, implementing policies and changes which directly affect the way in which nurses are able (or unable) to work, but who hardly ever talk to them. I know of a nursing assistant who had worked in the hospital for two years and yet the senior nurse manager did not even know what her name was or what she did. Those very managers who offer nothing in terms of support or encouragement; nothing in terms of help or advice, are the same managers who are only too pleased to jump on any nurse who steps out of line; the same managers who were once themselves practising nurses. And, of course, they believe it was all so much better in their day, that standards have dropped. There are managers who seem to be more interested in the nurses' dress sense than in their ability to deliver high quality humanitarian care. These days it's all about image. All about how we are perceived rather than what we are like and what we do. There is so much mutual mistrust, suspicion and paranoia that it makes any kind of practical working relationship almost impossible. Managers implement unpopular policies and nurses do everything in their power covertly to subvert them; to bend the rules and get away with things. It's like being at school again, except that those involved are supposed to be adults. One example that springs to mind is the no-smoking policy. Being an organisation concerned with health and health promotion, its staff cannot be seen to be indulging in behaviours which are bad for health. What would people think? So they introduce a no-smoking policy and the nurses who do smoke, do it in the toilets or around the back of the ward out of sight — just like smoking in the bike sheds at school. The nurses moan and complain about virtually everything — poor pay; poor conditions; stress; the attitudes of doctors, managers, relatives and the patients themselves who are often demanding, difficult and emotionally draining. Yet nowhere in any of this does there appear to be anything constructive being done. There seems to be no viable resolution for any of these problems. Instead, there is stalemate and hopelessness. You either accept things the way they are, or you get out. I've seen many good nurses leave simply because they just cannot stick it any more. Often it is the best nurses who leave to move elsewhere.

Most nurses are familiar with the new notions of empowerment (Rodwell, 1996) both for nurses and for the patients who suffer most from this mess. And, because this has become the established way, they treat these new notions with the same mix of suspicion and apathy, with which they treat nearly everything else: 'Nothing is going to change. It never has, so why get all excited about the latest in a long line of great ideas?' Nurses have been used to a long history of disempowerment; of being the underdog, of being ineffective, unappreciated and down-trodden. The nurse academics, sitting in their ivory towers, write endlessly about the potential for the nursing 'profession' — some with a degree of scepticism (Porter, 1992) — but most nurses that I know have never read anything they write. Whenever I talk about this sort of thing, which I do rarely and with a large degree of trepidation, other nurses look at me as if I have just arrived from another planet and have no appreciation of the real world at all. Of course I do, because like them I work in it every day. Our world is one of working, working as a nurse and all that it entails. For them, however, one of the things that nursing does *not* entail is the act of opposing or calling into question. Rather, it is about following the established norms; working in a way which has been brought about through years of nursing history, and following the rules which have been set.

Of course, this reaction is something borne out of experience. Nursing has undergone many, many years of disempowerment. Nurses have always been the subordinates, the juniors, the ones expected to do whatever is asked of them whether or not they agree.

This is a way of life that the 'profession' has got used to and it is now accepted as the norm. Those in the universities and colleges, and those within nursing who have the ambition of raising the status of the occupation — of possibly making it the equal of medicine — are really up against it. It is going to take a major shift in the thinking of all nurses. If those attempting to change the situation are contending with the established way of things and are unable to change them, then they are surely doomed to fail.

Do we have to accept the view that there is little prospect of change for nursing? There is a new breed of nurse entering the fray (Porter, 1994). In recent years, nursing has been trying to establish the 'critical nurse', the thinker; one who is able to examine particular issues related to nursing practice, whether they be patient-related or otherwise. Such nurses would not accept norms, but would question them: Why are they there? What purpose do they serve? Can they be changed? How? Hope, therefore, has not entirely disappeared. Nursing has got a chance of overcoming some, if not all, of the major obstacles which confront it. The future would appear to hold a number of areas of optimism. My major concern is that nurses of the future will have to fight the history of nursing — how it is expected that nurses should behave, how they should be. Once again, we are back to the issue of power. The question which I still have, is as follows: Will the 'new nurses' have the ability to bring about the changes which the whole 'profession', I am sure, would certainly desire — their freedom, their liberation, and their equality in a highly disempowering health service?

Points for reflection

The following issues were raised within this chapter:

1. Challenging authority as a newly-qualified practitioner.
2. The role of the critical thinker within nursing.
3. The relationship between theory and practice in caring.

References

Brewer AM, Lok P (1995) Managerial strategies and nursing commitment in Australian hospitals. *J Adv Nurs* **21**: 789–99

Cheek J, Rudge T (1993) The power of normalisation: Foucauldian perspectives on contemporary Australian health care practices. *Aust J Social Issues* **28** (4): 271–84

Conway J (1994) Reflection, the art and science of nursing and the theory practice gap. *Br J Nurs* **3**(3) : 114–8

Department of Health (1983) *Mental Health Act.* HMSO, London

Gabe J, Calnan M, Bury M (1991) *The Sociology of the Health Service.* London, Routledge

Porter S (1992) The poverty of professionalization: a critical analysis of strategies for the occupational advancement of nursing. *J Adv Nurs* **17**: 720–6

Porter S (1993) The determinants of psychiatric nursing practice: a comparison of sociological perspectives. *J Adv Nurs* **18**: 1559–66

Porter S (1994) New nursing: the road to freedom? *J Adv Nurs* **20**: 269–74

Rodwell C (1996) An analysis of the concept of empowerment. *J Adv Nurs* **23**: 305–13

UKCC (1992) *Professional Code of Conduct.* UKCC, London

Walsh M, Ford P (1989) *Nursing rituals: research and rational action.* Heinemann, Oxford

Warner C (1992) Responding to aggression. *Nurs Times* **88** (30): 46–7

4

Ageing and empowerment: Questions and dilemmas

Ian Stuart-Hamilton

Introduction

It would be easy to present this chapter as a hymn of praise to empowerment in older people. Nobody doubts that it is in principle a 'good thing', and the rest of this chapter could consist of an uncritical eulogy to this effect. However, this would miss a fundamental point. Although empowerment *per se* is undoubtedly good, it must be seen against a background of extensive research on other, related topics. These place empowerment in a different light — not necessarily unflattering, but certainly one indicating the need for caution and, indeed, pessimism in use. To demonstrate this point, we will begin by considering a single case study of self-empowerment. We will then consider the general issue of empowerment in later life before searching for the root causes of this in studies of psychological and social change in older people.

Our first consideration is the case study of an individual which will be used to illuminate some of the theoretical concerns about the issue of empowerment. It is customary in cases of empowerment to cite instances of triumph overcoming adversity. There are sound reasons for doing this, but it can become a little wearying to present all cases of ageing as examples of problems waiting to be overcome. The following case presents an individual who has, to all intents and purposes, always been in tune with his ageing.

A case study with Alan

At the time of writing, Alan is sixty-five years old. As he himself acknowledges his lifestyle, though superficially different, in many ways repeats that of his father, Tom. The latter led a physically active life — a keen tennis player, he gradually cut back on participating in the sport as it became too demanding physically (though he still played a fairly gentle game into his late seventies), taking up cycling and then walking. Gardening, which he had loved throughout his life, was an activity in which he could engage right up until his final months. This last period was one during which Tom came to terms with his lot. He had arranged his will, he knew death was imminent and announced it without fear, and he finally died having made peace with all who knew him. There are worse epitaphs.

As a child, Alan attempted racket sports but, unlike his father, was 'cheerfully hopeless' at them. However, he enjoyed running and, relatively unusually for one of his generation, continued to run for exercise and enjoyment after he left school. His membership of the local athletics club was used more for the facilities and the opportunities to run than for the social concerns, and running continued as a key interest throughout his middle age. Pressure of work prevented the hobby from being taken very seriously (before retirement, Alan was a successful commercial artist — several famous charity and commercial logos are his designs) until the encroachment of early old age. At about this time, triathlon was becoming recognised as a sport (for the uninitiated, this is a race comprising a long swim, a long bike ride and then a long run with no break in between the activities). Triathlon captured Alan's imagination and he began to enter competitions. At the age of sixty, his performance was sufficiently good for him to be selected for the British senior men's team at the world championships, in which he obtained a creditable middle ranking. He has since represented his country internationally on other occasions.

Alan's competitive triathlete days may be numbered, however. He has contracted a painful heel spur which makes running difficult, although he still cycles and swims at a 'serious' level of training. Faced with the question of what he will do if the injury permanently prevents him from running, Alan is phlegmatic. Yes, of course he will miss running but he realises that if the heel spur does not bar him from running, then other age-related factors eventually will. However, the purpose of running is to help to keep him fit and active, and there are other ways in which these goals can be attained. The same applies to cycling and swimming — they are, of course, enjoyable, but they are a means to an end. Indeed, the trappings of success at sport are kept modestly hidden, with trophies and so on kept tucked away in his home office and not on full view in the drawing room. For once, the cliché about not winning but taking part seems apt.

Pressing him further on the issue of adjusting to changing circumstances, I asked Alan what he would do if all triathlon activities became impossible. 'Then,' he replied happily, 'I would concentrate on walking.' (His wife is a keen rambler, and Alan and she go on walking holidays.) Probing, I asked what he would do if some awful accident prevented walking? 'Then,' replied Alan, 'I would do more painting.' (As a retired commercial artist, there is a feeling of wanting to paint all the uncommercial topics business sense had prevented.) What if he became quadriplegic? Then he would try to grip a paintbrush in his teeth. Alan elaborated on this theme. He felt that everyone is given a certain level of skill and must try to attain what he or she can at that level. Over time, abilities will gradually decrease, but it is just as great an accomplishment to meet the new standards as it was to meet earlier ones. Alan has a clearly-delineated life plan in which there are well-defined and realistic goals (very akin to those of his father but, though Alan acknowledges the similarities, he denies deliberate copying). Few would dispute that he is adequately self-empowered.

Alan's case is, of course, extreme. Few of us are, or will become, international athletes. However, that is not the point of the case study. Rather, it is to portray a person who attained what was realisable for himself. There is little doubt amongst those who know him that had his highest possible accomplishment been to win an egg-and-spoon race at a village fete, then the satisfaction would have been the same. The attainment of realistic ability-appropriate goals is, therefore, a clear example of how empowerment can be attained and reinforced. However, what is left out of Alan's life story is just as revealing as what is contained within it. For example, it would be fair to state that he has a relatively small circle of friends. This is not to say that Alan is in any way an unfriendly or inhospitable person — far from it. However, his emotional nutrition has tended to come from his immediate family, his work and his running. There is nothing 'wrong' with this, but it demonstrates that many other people, for whom an active social life is far more important, would not find Alan's lifestyle empowering. Concentrating on rewarding activities, and adjusting these according to circumstances, would not be a viable solution. If one's whole life has been spent enjoying social activity, how does one compensate adequately for a loss of human company? There are, of course, methods available but here the need for skilled and sympathetic intervention becomes clearer. Indeed, extrapolating from this point, it is apparent that for a person to remain self-empowered, the less other people are needed, the better. If a person relies upon attainable goals which can be afforded and are available, then self-empowerment is possible, but relying on the presence of others cannot be so easily guaranteed.

This creates a rather bleak view of empowerment in spite of a superficially optimistic air. Empowerment may be necessary, but the degree of need is tempered by the needs of the individual. Although an easy rule of thumb is impossible, it might tentatively be suggested that empowerment is most likely to succeed when it only needs to provide little support. The more it has to provide, and the more this relies upon other people, the less likely it is to succeed.

Empowerment and ageing

The general literature concerning empowerment presents a similarly guarded view of the subject. It is undoubtedly true that it is a good and useful thing in appropriate circumstances. For example, Mok and Mui (1996) report its successful use in improving the well-being of the residents in a retirement home. It is interesting to note that the researchers also demonstrated clearly to the home's staff that the empowerment also aided themselves, and was not a threat to their professional functioning (cf Sharpe, 1995). Indeed, it is difficult to find any arguments against empowerment *per se* in the literature. However, there are many reservations expressed about the extent of its effectiveness. Perhaps the most common is the question of who controls the empowerment — if an individual has to be shown how to be empowered by someone else, is this true empowerment, or patronage? The question may at first strike the reader as ridiculous: no one, for example, would claim that Einstein had not 'properly' attained eminence simply because as a child he had to be taught mathematics. So why should the provenance of an individual's empowerment matter? However, in certain cases, older people (and their caregivers) may feel incapable of acting without the permission or (in complex cases) advice of professionals. In such instances, providing empowerment becomes a gift to be bestowed by an 'expert', and one which further increases the sense of control which the healthcare professional has over the older person (Brown and Furstenberg, 1992).

Healthcare professionals tread a thin line. Not only must they be wary of offering empowerment, but they must also be wary of taking it away (albeit for the best of intentions). For example, Beckingham and Watt (1995) note that, in trying to help older people who have fallen ill, any attempts to restrict 'unhealthy' activities may be interpreted as disempowerment and a general restriction of freedom. This raises a further knotty problem about empowerment. We have already noted that the term will mean different things to different people. In addition, it must now be noted that a withdrawal of power may in some cases be necessary for an individual's own good. And, as with the discussion above, there is no easy solution to this problem; no simple utilitarian formula to be applied in all cases. Restricting freedom is always a dangerous step, but in some cases it is best for all concerned, even if it is not appreciated at the time. This smacks dangerously of 'Nanny knows best' — or worse, but as with all healthcare, some pragmatism is always needed.

However, the caveats to be attached to empowerment do not simply end with the problems of when to offer it and the personalities of the recipients. For example, ethnic grouping is likely to shape demand characteristics and perceived areas of strength and weakness (Zimmerman *et al*, 1992).

The list could be prolonged, but the point has surely been made — there are so many caveats that it is difficult to make blanket statements about the 'correct' form which empowerment should take. Indeed, no one in the literature on ageing seems sure about what the outcome of 'successful' empowerment should be. We may have a vague idea that people should be in charge of their own lives. In some respects, this is good news. For example, a lowering of the burden on the caring professions resulting from people taking greater care of their own welfare makes economic sense. However, by the same token, so also does voluntary euthanasia. Again, of course, being empowered does not necessarily mean being 'happy'. There are many different personality types and, for some, the concept of contentment is indeed synonymous with empowerment. Others, however, are more likely to be happy only if lacking the very empowerment which others crave. What is right for Alan may be hopelessly wrong for another individual with, for example, a more sedentary lifestyle revolving around parties and other social events. Baltes (1996) demonstrates that the optimal level of responsibility and social interaction will vary markedly both between individuals and within individuals across the lifespan. Whilst it is fair to say that no one should be allowed to abnegate all responsibility, a wish to let some things be decided on one's behalf is a sensible one (at any age), and any attempts to empower such people 'too much' will meet with justifiable resentment and unhappiness. By the same token, as we have just seen, it may be appropriate to lessen the power of some individuals who would prefer more. It is thus true to say that each individual will have an optimal level of empowerment. What this is can only be discovered on an individual basis: no easily-applied rule can or should be inflicted. However, this does not mean that we should not be aware of the issues involved. This, in turn, begs the question: What factors create the need for empowerment and why will it differ between individuals? To answer this, we need to take a step back and consider the general questions of psychological ageing and self-image.

Defining ageing

The concept of 'ageing' is surprisingly nebulous. The first problem concerns what is meant by 'age'. Chronological age (that is, how many times the Earth has been around the Sun since one's birth) is the traditional measure, but it is only a guide to other states. For example, people aged sixty years can differ enormously from each other in terms of physical and mental state. Everyday experience shows that we consider some individuals as being 'young' or 'old' 'for their age'. Therefore, a 'typical' person of a particular age is only an approximation, with room for considerable differences between the actual members of an age group. One needs only to consider the example of Alan and compare him with a prototypical man of the same age to see the considerable range possible. Indeed, the evidence indicates that the older the age group considered, the greater the spread of variability. In other words, the older the group, the more unrepresentative the 'average' becomes (Stuart-Hamilton, 1994).

A further problem which arises concerns what is meant by the terms 'old age' or 'ageing'. In a very general sense, the meaning is clear — it is a change over time. However, in that sense, an individual growing from baby to child could be said to be 'ageing'. At one level this is, of course, true but intuitively we feel that the term is being used inappropriately. Instead, we are more inclined to accept the term when it is reserved for describing changes which occur in later adult life. Generally, researchers and practitioners adopt a rule of thumb that 'old age' begins at a person's sixtieth birthday (Stuart-Hamilton, 1994). There are sound pragmatic reasons for dividing the lifespan into conceptual units, but one pays a price and, in the case of ageing, it is a heavy one. The biggest mental and physical changes occur in childhood and in the final years of life.

Because the former ends in adulthood and the latter in death, a contrast is established which practically guarantees that ageing is seen first and foremost in terms of decay. Empowerment is thus compromised by a mental schema which casts ageing, at best, in an unflattering light and, at worst, as a blind prejudice. The reality of ageing is that it is far more capricious and resistant to objective measurement, which creates an ironic counterpoint. This can be proven by considering the supposed 'decline' in psychological powers, such as intelligence.

Ageing and intelligence

It is certainly true that if one takes the average intelligence or memory test scores for different adult age groups, then there is a statistically significant decline in people aged sixty years and over (for example, Salthouse, 1991). However, this change is not valid for everybody within an age group. Indeed, about fifteen per cent of older adults will retain the level of intellectual/memory performance which they have always possessed (Stuart-Hamilton, 1994). Amongst the remainder, at least part of the difference in performance between older and younger adults will not be due to ageing as such, but to peripheral factors such as the increased physical frailty of the older respondents (Salthouse, 1991). For example, many older adults write less quickly because of muscular and joint problems. This will obviously be disadvantageous in paper and pencil intelligence tests where answers must be written down as quickly as possible. Indeed, one researcher, Storandt (1976, 1977), calculated that as much as half of the difference between younger and older adults may be due to differences in speed of writing rather than to thought *per se*. In other words, a large part of 'ageing decline' may be a product of how we choose to measure it. This leads us to a discussion of the cohort effect. A difference in performance between two adult age groups may be due to their age difference, but equally the two groups have been educated and brought up in radically different ways (for example, compare the first two decades of a person born in 1930 with those of someone born in 1960). Therefore, the difference could be as much a matter of upbringing as of the supposed effects of 'ageing decay'. One way round this problem is to adopt a longitudinal study in which the same people are tested both when young and when old (and hence any differences are supposedly due only to ageing, since the effects of any differences in upbringing have obviously been removed). Such studies tend to find age group differences, but they are less dramatic than when a conventional age group comparison is performed (Stuart-Hamilton, 1994).

This means that empowerment is compromised by a belief that older people 'must' be getting feeble minded, which is a fiction. There are ways of avoiding this trap. In the case of Alan and similar people, a dedication to a chosen hobby may mean that sitting back and thinking about how they are decaying is simply not an option they have thought of. Other groups may not take quite such a cavalier attitude, and see even the slightest change as a harbinger of 'senility'. It is ironic that often people may fret about such things using the very same intellectual powers that they have always had. Overall, it is certainly true that many people regard later life as a period of decline (Stuart-Hamilton, 1994, 1998), leading to guidelines about how older people 'should' behave which are usually not justified by the evidence. Societal norms are nearly always disempowering, and those concerning ageing are no exception.

Social ageing

There are powerful societal norms of acceptable behaviour for each particular chronological age group (often called the 'social age'). Everybody has a set of ideas about what a typical person of a particular age group should be like. These can be based on sound principles. For example, societal pressures are against children driving, drinking or having sex because they are activities not considered appropriate for their level of maturity. This is implicit in the phrase 'under age', and such a concept is not under serious criticism. With older people, such social age judgements can also be sensible. For example, older people are generally discouraged from taking part in physically dangerous sports such as bungee jumping, if for no other reason than that their bones are more brittle and mend less well. Even this stricture, however, cannot be followed too rigidly. The statement that a sixty-year-old man should not consider participating in triathlons might be taken at face value by many people until confronted with a case such as Alan's.

However, other rulings, even at face value, smack of little more than small town puritanism. The 'correct' behaviour of an older person can be seen in terms of a set of prescriptive activities which largely involve being sedentary (dispensing wisdom and generally not being a nuisance) and a (larger) set of prohibitions (essentially avoiding anything which 'should' be the preserve of younger adults). Again, the case study above rubbishes this point. More generally, many instances could be taken, but a particularly vivid point is made by restrictions on sexual behaviour. The idea of an active sex life for an older person is stereotypically considered disgusting by many people. Before readers begin to suppose 'perfectly true, but it doesn't apply to me', consider the following concepts:

A the marriage of a black man and a white woman
B the marriage of a sixty-year-old man and a twenty-year-old woman

It is sincerely hoped that the first statement causes no concern for readers. However, how many readers' first thoughts on reading concept B were something along the lines of 'dirty old man' or 'she must be after his money'? Alternatively, what if statement B had been describing the marriage of a sixty-year-old woman and a twenty-year-old man? What are the first thoughts which spring to mind? Some sound practical arguments can be produced against relationships with a large age difference (probably very different interests, the problems with raising children, a lengthy period of widowhood, and so on), but it is unlikely that these were high on the list of thoughts. Instead, there seems to be a deep-rooted antipathy against older people stepping outside the boundaries of what a particular society considers to be age-appropriate behaviour. Of course, things can change as, for example, has been shown in the case of racial and sexual discrimination. Only a few decades ago, the concept of a 'mixed marriage' as described in concept A above, would have caused outrage in most sections of the community. Today, such hostility would be considered unusual (and rightly so).

It is possible to draw out the analogy between racism and ageism further and to point out the considerable similarities between the forms of prejudice found in each case. This can be useful in highlighting the irrationality behind much of ageism and, indeed, as has been observed by many authors, a good rule of thumb is to substitute 'black' for 'old' in a statement to judge if it is prejudicial (Stuart-Hamilton, 1994). However, the analogy breaks down on two important issues. Firstly, the evidence against black or other racial minority groups was often based upon spurious 'scientific' evidence, such as (supposedly) statistically significantly lower IQ scores. However, as has been seen, the evidence of lower IQ scores is, alas, true for the average older person. Again, older people are generally less physically capable and are more likely to have a debilitating physical condition. Secondly, the case for racial equality is one which, on a priori grounds, is made for all social situations. The case for age equality is rather more specific. For example, older people are not generally concerned about equal employment opportunities or educational access. A simple summary is not possible but, in essence, the case is rather more about the need for recognition as an equal voice in situations where contact is made with others.

In the case study, Alan does not feel lack of status. He has proven himself in an area of endeavour which younger adults would find (literally) impossible to achieve. However, it is doubtful that, even if he had done nothing more strenuous than gardening, Alan would feel disempowered, because his strength comes from the achievement of personal goals rather than from comparisons with others or with social norms (indeed, it might be argued that he is actively defying norms, though he probably would not recognise this consciously). However, not everyone is in the fortunate position of Alan, and a feeling of lack of status has obvious implications for empowerment. If X feels less competent than Y, how can X claim to have the same dignity and right to respect as Y? However, whilst such arguments may be theoretically sound, what is the practical evidence on the status of older adults?

Self-image and ageing

Such equality of recognition is lacking, as even a cursory glance at the literature reveals. This is most evident from research on the perceived status of, and self-image in, older people. First, it can be established that negative feelings about older people are strongly held, more so even than stereotypes about gender differences (Kite *et al*, 1993). This problem is compounded by the finding that people perceive later life as a time when things will inevitably get worse, whereas other 'low status' groups (for example, children) are viewed as having the opportunity to improve (Ryff, 1991). Given such findings, it is not surprising that many older people feel a lowered self-image. A telling example of this is the avoidance of 'explicit' terms such as 'old' or 'aged' when older adults are asked to describe themselves (Ward, 1984). It is also pertinent to note that self-image is lower in elderly people who believe most strongly in stereotypes (Ward, 1977). In other words, if one spends younger adulthood fervently believing in the dreadful nature of 'old age', then one is doomed to become the very stereotype one despised (there is an element of poetic justice in this, but it is only likely to be savoured by those with a particular taste for *schadenfreude*). The problem with negative stereotypes of older people is thus twofold. Aside from the harm they cause older people, they also will ultimately harm many of those who hold them. Ageism is a unique prejudice in that it is the only one where the hater has a good chance of becoming the hated. Disempowerment can be self-inflicted.

However, it is important to note that the problem of poor self-image can be overplayed. Whilst it is right and proper that we should be concerned about ageism and its effects, it is very easy to slip into portraying older people purely as victims. This, of course, only further reinforces the negative image (albeit for the best of intentions). It also creates an atmosphere in which it is easy to imagine that the only way in which empowerment can occur is by being bestowed by a member of the caring professions and that older people, if unaided by younger adults, must inevitably be miserable and stuck in a lower caste. However, findings of lowered image can be exaggerated by the way in which studies have presented their questions. Usually, questions about the status of older people are made in a manner inviting direct comparison with younger adults, or in conjunction with a consideration of a typical older person's financial state. Neither method is likely to create a roseate glow of contentment about later life. However, if adults are asked about later life without explicit comparisons being invited, then opinions from all age groups are more positive, and even optimistic (Stuart-Hamilton, 1998). Thus, the extent to which we wish to see older people as having a poor self-image, or younger adults having negative views about older, may in part depend upon how we ask the question.

Personality and ageing

Empowerment fits into a rather more complex picture than might at first be imagined. It cannot be seen as a gift to be bestowed by healthcare professionals and social workers on a poor, defenceless, elderly population who would otherwise, inevitably, be crushed under a weight of oppressive societal forces, fading abilities and self-doubt. Not all will need it, and for those who do, reasons (and hence responses) may be various. This final point is supported by the findings about the various personality types and preferred lifestyles of older people (Perlmutter and Hall, 1992). The stereotype of all older adults being hostile and complaining is, of course, a myth. Some individuals will be like this, but the likelihood is that they were similarly unpleasant in their earlier life. The adult personality is reasonably unvarying through the lifespan, and it would be wrong to blame ageing for every disagreeable personality trait (for example, Perlmutter and Hall, 1992; Stuart-Hamilton, 1994).

Researchers from a variety of backgrounds have examined personality in late adulthood, and each has devised his or her own particular classificatory system. Arguably, common to all is a judgement of the extent to which the individual is at peace with himself or herself and the world. The greater the serenity, the more 'successful' the personality type. Amongst the best known of such measures is Erikson's (1982) concept of ego integration, which argues that the final stage of life should see an attainment of acceptance and a tying-up of 'loose ends'.

Other researchers from rather different theoretical backgrounds can be argued to have said the same thing, though this is not surprising since few would argue that a life of inner turmoil and neuroticism is a good thing. If we consider the literature concerning the lifestyles of older people, then we find that, generally, those considered to be most successful are also those most at peace. For example, in Neugarten *et al*'s (1961, 1968) celebrated studies, four principal personality types (with subdivisions) were identified. The most desirable type was the integrated personality (subdivided into: reorganisers — as one activity became physically impossible, then another was found; focused — activities were limited to a small set of feasible and highly rewarding ones; and disengaged — the deliberate abnegation of many responsibilities). Alan is arguably a very good example of an integrated personality. He is currently focused on a small band of activities, but his future plans reveal him to be a reorganiser. There are clear indicators that he will always attempt to concentrate on some form of activity and, if triathlons become impossible, other less physically demanding pursuits will be taken up in their place. Another major Neugarten trait (though less satisfactory than the integrated type) was the armoured-defensive personality (divided into: holding on — staving off decay by maintaining a high level of activity; and constricted — dwelling on what had been lost as a result of ageing). A third group was labelled passive-dependent and characterised by a reliance on others for many needs. A fourth and final group comprised the disorganised personalities, where there was clear evidence of abnormal (and dementing?) functioning. There have been other categorisations of personality types in later life (for example, Butcher *et al*, 1991; Neugarten, 1977; Thomas, 1980), but all are in general agreement that there are different responses to ageing and no single type describes everyone.

It therefore follows from this that empowerment is likely to mean very different things to different people and, indeed, that some groups of older people may resent attempts at personal empowerment. For example, it is most unlikely that Neugarten's passive-dependent personalities (Reichard *et al*, 1962 found a similar group and called them 'rocking chair personalities') would welcome attempts to make them more responsible and in control of their own lives. This raises the question of whether healthcare professionals 'should' encourage empowerment if an individual clearly does not want it. Pushed too far, such an argument begins to sound like the reasoning for a disengagement theory, but the fact remains that not everyone wants power, so should it be thrust upon them? However, given dwindling economic resources, there is a utilitarian case in favour of making individuals help themselves as much as possible, thus liberating resources for other things (cf Lloyd, 1991). It would be possible to continue this debate for several more pages without gaining further ground in either direction. Which side one supports ultimately depends upon the pragmatics of each individual situation — there is no obvious blanket statement which can cover all occasions when such a decision needs to be made. Indeed, authors writing about empowerment in older people often remark upon the importance of addressing the specific context of each problem (Perkinson, 1992; Scheidt and Norris-Baker, 1993). However, a point has been made — namely that empowerment is not automatically a good thing.

Conclusions

In general, later life is characterised by a decline in intellectual and memory skills, and in perceived status. This is the primary fuel for disempowerment and is, naturally, a cause for concern. Firstly, because it acts against a priori feelings of natural equality and secondly, because in any case, many of the supposed age-related changes are artifacts of the experiments and measures used. In other words, seeing later life as a perfect synonym of decline is erroneous. The case study of Alan vividly illustrates that later life need not be a time of physical decline (indeed, Alan is arguably physically fitter than most younger adults) and that even if decline does strike, it need not be disempowering.

However, we need to be very careful in being too enthusiastic about empowerment. Older people may, by nature of their intellect and/or personality, be optimally served by abnegating responsibility for a greater or lesser proportion of their lives. Regarding everyone as needing an equal amount of simple 'power' is counter-productive and ultimately patronising. But how does one create the right level for an individual? This places the health professional on the horns of a dilemma: remove the right of choice from the individual to too great an extent, and the individual is not only losing self-empowerment, but is being made to function at a level below their abilities. This is both inefficient and, more importantly, arguably reduces self-image. However, bestowing too much responsibility on a person may be creating an irksome load, which is stretching an individual beyond their means and, hence, is once again inefficient and will create a lowering of self-image because the person cannot cope. The picture is further muddied when one considers that what is a source of empowerment for one person will be a source of disempowerment for another. Thus, in our case study, the physical activities and the relatively solitary life of Alan is fed upon factors which would be anathema to a more sedentary person. Empowerment must ultimately be unique to each individual.

Points for reflection

The following issues were raised within this chapter:

1. Empowerment is not automatically a good thing for the elderly client.
2. Society's norms may well disempower the elderly client.
3. There are a variety of forms of empowerment.
4. Self-empowerment is possible for the elderly client.

References

Baltes M (1996) *The Many Faces of Dependency in Old Age.* Cambridge University Press, Cambridge

Beckingham AC, Watt S (1995) Daring to grow old: Lessons in healthy ageing and empowerment. *Educational Gerontol* **21**: 479–95

Brown JS, Furstenberg AL (1992) Restoring control: Empowering older patients and their families during health crises. *Soc Work Health Care* **17**: 81–101

Butcher JN, Aldwin CM, Levenson MR, *et al* (1991) Personality and ageing: A study of the MMPI-2 among older men. *Psychol Ageing* **6**: 361–70

Erikson EH (1982) *The Life Cycle Completed: a Review.* Norton, New York

Kite ME, Deaux K, Miele M (1993) Stereotypes of young and old: Does age outweigh gender? *Psychol Ageing* **8**: 19–27

Lloyd P (1991) The empowerment of elderly people. *J Ageing Studies* **5**: 125–35

Mok B, Mui A (1996) Empowerment in residential care for the elders: The case of an aged home in Hong Kong. *J Gerontological Soc Work* **27**: 23–35

Neugarten BL (1977) Personality and ageing. In: Birren JE, Schaie KW eds *Handbook of the Psychology of Ageing.* Reinhold, New York

Neugarten BL, Havinghurst RJ, Tobin SS (1961) The measurement of life satisfaction. *J Gerontol* **16** 134–43.

Neugarten BL, Havinghurst RJ, Tobin SS (1968) Personality and pattern of ageing. In: Neugarten BL ed *Middle Age and Ageing.* Chicago University Press, Chicago

Perkinson MA (1992) Maximizing personal efficacy in older adults: The empowerment of volunteers in a multipurpose senior center. *Phys Occup Ther Geriatr* **10:** 57–72

Perlmutter M, Hall E (1992) *Adult Development and Ageing.* John Wiley, New York

Reichard S, Livson F, Peterson PG (1962) *Ageing and personality: A study of 87 older men.* Wiley, New York

Ryff CD (1991) Possible selves in adulthood and old age: A tale of shifting horizons. *Psychol Ageing* **6**: 286–95

Salthouse TA (1991) *Theoretical Perspectives on Cognitive Ageing.* Erlbaum, Hillsdale, New Jersey

Scheidt RJ, Norris-Baker C (1993) The environmental context of poverty among older residents of economically endangered Kansas towns. *J Appl Gerontol* **12**: 335–48

Sharpe PA (1995) Older women and health services: Moving from ageism toward empowerment. *Women and Health* **22:** 9–23

Storandt M (1976) Speed and coding effects in relation to age and ability level. *Dev Psychol* **12**: 177–8.

Storandt M (1977) Age, ability level and scoring the WAIS. *J Gerontol* **32**: 175–8

Stuart-Hamilton I (1994) *The Psychology of Ageing. An Introduction.* 2nd edn, Jessica Kingsley Publishers, London

Stuart-Hamilton I (1998) Women's attitudes to ageing: some factors of relevance to educational gerontology. *Educ Ageing* **13**: 67–88

Thomas H (1980) Personality and adjustment to ageing. In: Birren JE, Sloane RB eds *Handbook of Mental Health and Ageing.* Prentice-Hall, New Jersey

Ward R (1977) The impact of subjective age and stigma on older persons. *J Gerontol* **32**: 227–32

Ward RA (1984) *The ageing experience.* Harper & Row, Cambridge

Zimmerman MA, Israel BA, Schulz AJ, *et al* (1992) Further explorations in empowerment theory: An empirical analysis of psychological empowerment. *Am J Community Psychol* **20**: 707–27

Part II

Empowerment through reflection: Making sense of practice

5

Empowerment through reflection: Is this a case of the emperor's new clothes?

Tony Ghaye

That wonderful children's fairy tale by Hans Christian Andersen called 'The emperor's new clothes', carries with it an unintended, yet important message for those who continue to promote the benefits of reflective practices in healthcare. One proclaimed benefit is that individuals and groups may well become empowered through reflection of one kind or another. In this chapter, I will be presenting some of the claims being made about reflective practices. This leads on to a discussion of the way empowerment is associated with the equally slippery notions of power and reality.

Many years ago, there was an emperor who was excessively fond of new clothes. Most of all he loved to show them off. One day, two swindlers came to town masquerading as weavers who could make the most beautiful clothes imaginable. Not only this, but these clothes had the magical quality of becoming invisible to all those who were not fit for the office they held, or who were impossibly dull. The emperor thought that these would be splendid clothes and so ordered some to be made for himself. He thought that by wearing them he would be able to discover those people in his kingdom who were unfit for their posts. He also thought he would be able to tell the wise men from the fools. The two swindlers pocketed much money in undertaking the work, pretending to weave and yet having nothing of substance on their shuttles. Soon, word spread and everyone came to know the claims being made about the wonderful powers the clothes possessed. Ministers and courtiers came and went. They could see nothing, but they took care not to say so. They did not wish to appear foolish or unfit for their posts. They watched and listened to the swindlers. When they were told to step nearer so that they might more fully appreciate the patterns and colouring in the emperor's new clothes, they did so dutifully and unquestioningly. When the emperor went to see for himself, even he was taken in. 'What,' thought the emperor, 'I see nothing at all! This is terrible! Am I a fool? Am I not fit to be an emperor?... Oh, it is beautiful!' he said. 'It has my highest approval.' And he nodded his satisfaction as he gazed at the empty loom. Nothing would induce him to say that he could not see anything. He was even persuaded to wear the new clothes for the occasion of a great procession which was about to take place.

On the day of the procession, the chamberlains pretended to lift and carry the emperor's cloak as he walked along under a gorgeous canopy. Everyone in the streets shouted, 'How beautiful the emperor's new clothes are! They fit to perfection, and what a splendid cloak!' Nobody would admit that they could see nothing. No one wanted either to be deemed unfit for their post, or to appear to be a fool.

'But he's got nothing on,' shouted a little boy.

'Oh, listen to the innocent!' said his father.

But then one person whispered to the other what the child had said: 'He's got nothing on! The child says he has nothing on!'

'But he has got nothing on!' all the people cried at last.

The emperor writhed and looked uncomfortable for he knew it was true. But he decided that the procession must go on. So he held his head up prouder than ever. His chamberlains continued to carry aloft the invisible cloak. The two swindlers were made 'gentlemen weavers' and selfishly put all the silk and gold thread into their own pockets.

This story gives us much to reflect upon. It describes different realities and, because of this, gives us some interesting insights into notions of empowerment. It also serves to remind us that it is dangerous to be swept along by any tide of events (including, perhaps, reflective practices) despite loud fanfares and much flag waving; that it can be very dangerous to receive others' 'wisdom' unquestioningly; that we should be able to make up our own minds about the value of things; that we should not be afraid to speak out, to 'go against the flow', to ask for evidence rather than blindly accepting 'reality' as described by others. There are links with reflection here. Reflective practices continue to gain ground. More and more resources are being devoted to its promotion. Libraries are being filled with texts about it. People's careers are being fashioned by it and conferences proclaim its centrality to improvement and lifelong learning in healthcare work and policy. There is much flag waving and some blind faith. In this chapter I aim to set out some of the claims being made for reflective practices. More particularly, I want to explore some of the claims being made that individuals and groups can become empowered through reflection. 'Empowerment' and 'reflection' are problematic in that they mean different things to different people. They are encountered in different ways. I intend here to focus on views of empowerment, because a whole book in this series (Ghaye and Lillyman, 2000) is devoted to the nature of reflection. In this chapter, I want to raise an important issue for your consideration. It is this: that despite all the efforts being made to foster empowerment through reflective practices, it remains very much like the emperor's new clothes. We speak about and celebrate it loudly in public and yet we may ask ourselves privately, 'Where is the evidence, from practice, to support such a celebration?' We might have private misgivings. We might ask: 'Why can't I see it when others say they can? Has it really led to some kind of transformation in healthcare? Whose reality is this? Whose reality counts?'

How far are reflective practices 'appealing'? A question of reality

In 1994, James and Clarke set out in a questioning way, what they regarded as the 'appeal' of reflective practice for nursing. For example, they claimed that:

> ***Reflection is an integral part of experiential learning and the development of practical knowledge.***
> *Much of the attraction of reflective practices is that reflection is firmly grounded in a growing understanding of forms of practical knowledge and of experiential learning. Reflection is central to many theories of experiential learning (Kolb, 1984), which is arguably the dominant form of learning in nursing. It is significant in the processes of learning in adults (Knowles 1970, Mezirow 1981) and it is the subject of an influential body of literature (Schon 1983, Benner 1984, Powell 1989). As such, at a fundamental level, models of reflective practice have an appeal because they ground that practice in established theory which can offer practitioners and practitioner educators frameworks in which to operate.*
>
> ***Reflection will lead to better practice.***
> *Implicit in the status currently being given to reflective practices in nursing, is an accepted view that reflection*

will lead to better practice and to greater competence. There is, in fact, little or no hard evidence for this assumption although, in time, research evidence may show this assumption to be correct.

Reflective practice is necessary for effective nursing.
There is an implicit assumption in the justification for adopting a reflective practice model of nursing that reflection is necessary for effective nursing. Again, there is no a priori justification for this and the case remains unproven, particularly with regard to reflection in the moral-ethical domain.

Reflective practice will bring universal benefits.
Even if we assume that reflection will produce benefits, it is most likely that not all of them will be equally acceptable to everyone. Improvements through reflection in efficiency at the technical level could be very attractive to those who are accountable in a managerial sense for a nurse's practice. However, the outcomes of reflection at other levels may not be so appealing for that group. Reflection at the moral-ethical level could result in many nurses coming to understand more clearly, through the development of self-knowledge in the emancipatory domain (Habermas, 1974), the everyday constraints and limitations placed upon their practice. These nurses could well begin to challenge those whom they see as responsible (that is, their managers) for exerting those constraints and limitations. A parallel issue may arise in the relationship between the student nurse and her or his educator.

All nurses can be reflective practitioners.
Although nurses require particular skills and qualities to become reflective, the message appears to be that all can acquire them. Those who are advocating a reflective practice model of nursing could usefully consider the implications for the profession if the notion that everyone can become a reflective practitioner proves not to be the case.

Reflective practice models enhance professional status.
Reflection and reflective practices may be attractive because they are seen increasingly as a central

> *characteristic of professional action. The emphasis in attempts to define an occupation as a profession has changed in recent years. It has broadened from concerns with the place and role of professions in society to encompass the nature of professional action. As professional practice becomes synonymous with reflective practices (see, for example, Schon, 1983), the use of reflective practitioner models of action could have some value in enhancing the professional status of nursing.*
>
> ***Reflective practices value each nurse's professional knowledge.***
> *Implicit in the concept of reflective practices is the valuing of each practitioner's own personal knowledge. As such, reflective practice models of nursing appear to value individual nursing practitioners and the contribution each of them has to offer. Reflective practices are apparently grounded in such 'high-level' values as democracy and equality and may, as a result, pose an attraction for many. A consequence of reflective practices is that nursing knowledge is not possessed by an élite group which has sole access to it; rather, all nurses hold their own theory of nursing. This could well have implications for the way nursing theory is conceptualised and generated.*
>
> (James and Clarke, 1994, pp.82–90)

What are some of the current claims being made for reflective practices? Whose reality? Whose fantasy?

Six years on, in the year 2000, we find ourselves in a situation where reflective practices have continued to gain ground both in the hearts, minds and practices of healthcare workers locally, and in implementing new government policy, such as clinical governance, throughout the National Health Service in the UK. As we begin the new millennium, there appear to be five broad claims being made for reflective practices. In general, they are claims which suggest that reflective practices are a good thing, that they make you feel good and that reflective practitioners make a positive difference in the clinical workplace. Some of these claims are more explicitly supported with evidence than others! I want, briefly, to set out the nature of these claims as I have come to understand them in the context of evidence-based practice and professionalism. It might be timely and prudent to 'test' the validity of each claim — we should not accept any claim uncritically. By so testing, we might move to a clearer conception of what reflective practices are and are not. I stress the plural term 'reflective practices' (see Ghaye and Lillyman, 2000) as there are many ways to reflect with practice in mind.

Claim 1: Reflective practices improve the quality of the care we give

- We can now more positively claim a link between reflection as personal and collective renewal and regeneration on the one hand, and improvements in the quality of action in practice on the other. For example, we can now find more examples of claims such as 'Reflective practice has transformed the work of …' (Rushton, 1999).
- These improvements can be known, valued and attributed to the processes of reflection-on-action.
- Becoming more reflective is increasingly being linked with the idea that the healthcare professional becomes a better practitioner. This is due to reflective practices forming a more explicit and secure part of our day-to-day work (Ghaye and Lillyman, 2000).

Claim 2: Reflective practices enhance individual and collective professional development

- The process of deepening our understanding and extending our professionalism is a consequence of reflecting on our clinical experiences.
- Reflective practices can help the healthcare worker to see more clearly and deeply. In this way, learning through reflection helps to develop confidence and competence. It can give us a greater sense of control over our own work. Some would go further and claim that reflective practices empower us. But what does this mean? Is this an over-claim? Does empowerment mean the confidence and ability to contest current healthcare trends, policies and practices? Does it mean the commitment, energy and capability to work collaboratively with significant others in conceiving, implementing and evaluating the impact of transformative healthcare action at the local, regional and

national level? Does empowerment mean being able to describe, explain and justify clinical practice when called upon to do so? Is empowerment through reflection a case of the emperor's new clothes? More about this later.
- Reflective practices can close the gap between what we say and what we do, and between our intentions and our achievements. In so doing, we gain a deeper understanding of the synchronicity and contradictions between our professional values and the workplace practices through which these values are expressed. It is, of course, a very difficult thing to be absolutely consistent. No one healthcare worker or NHS Trust ever is. It is difficult not to be a 'living contradiction' (Whitehead, 1993).

Claim 3: Reflective practices change the 'power' relationship between academics and practitioners by broadening who generates and controls knowledge for safe and competent healthcare

- Knowledge is not simply acquired from outside, taken on board, transferred and applied to the clinical environment; it is also acquired through critical reflections on practice. We can caricature this process as taking sole power and control away from one group, which we might generally call the academics or 'academy' representing the positivistic-bourgeois research tradition, in order to acknowledge that healthcare practitioners themselves have the power and right to control the processes of knowledge production and consumption.
- In addition to the principal modes through which the nursing profession has historically acquired knowledge — namely through tradition, authority, borrowing, trial and error, role modelling and mentorship (Ghaye *et al*, 1996), we can now legitimately add another. That is, the personal, practical knowledge acquired through reflective practices.
- The knowledge generated through reflective practices is knowledge generated to improve the *lebenswelt* (that is, the world of everyday life).

Claim 4: Reflective practices improve the clinical environment

- Reflective practice may not only improve individual and group work but can also transform the practice area in the medium and long term.

- Reflective practitioners should not ignore the 'structures' which condition their practice. Only by being 'critical' of them can the improvement process take a hold. The structures are embedded in the practical and micro-world of each of us. They are right there in front of us, every day, as we strive to give quality care to make the lives of the sick, aged, mentally ill, disabled and other groups more worthwhile, dignified and fulfilling.

Claim 5: Reflective practices help to build a better world

- Reflective practices not only connect with the 'local', immediate and that which is directly, right now, within our sphere of influence. They can also connect with hopes, intentions and struggles for more just, democratic, compassionate, caring and dignified healthcare systems.

In order for these claims to acquire more acceptance and credibility, there are perhaps five areas in which we might place more effort and questioning attention. The first is concerned with recent emphasis on evidence-based practice (McSherry and Haddock, 1999). Here we need to be very clear about what we mean by 'evidence', and which evidence is most appropriate to illuminate and resolve particular kinds of problems.

Secondly, and as a consequence of this, we need to clarify the different and fundamental interests and value positions of reflective practices. Who holds them? Where do they come from and why? Are the interests to do with personal renewal and development and/or with producing knowledge which can be applied to practice? Are the interests associated with solving healthcare problems, with understanding the life worlds of healthcare workers and clients and/or to do with organisational change? Are the interests essentially individualistic and private and/or to do with collective workplace learning where:

> *...workplace knowledge production means participation in the praxis of intervention and construction of new ways of working and new working goals, and in the formulation of more complex and sophisticated ways of valuing work, work culture and its place in people's lifeworlds.*
>
> (McTaggart, 1994, pp.320–1)

What other interests might reflective practices serve? There are many. Individual and collective empowerment, for example?

Thirdly, I believe we need to have a much greater discussion about the ontological, epistemological and methodological aspects of the processes of reflective practices within healthcare, and to link these discourses to issues of trustworthiness, authenticity and usefulness.

Fourthly, more attention needs to be given to the nature and potency of the theories-of-action which can arise from reflections-on-practice. This is not simply a case of trying to make 'theory' more practical or practice more 'theoretical', with the hope that this will improve healthcare. Our practices and the values they embody need to be made explicit.

Finally, the way reflective practices interrelate with the notion of collaborative practitioner research needs to be discussed more widely and shared.

So, how do these claims link to understandings of empowerment? A question of multiple realities

The word 'empowerment' crops up a great deal in healthcare. There is no universally agreed definition of it. As soon as we get into the literature on empowerment we find that it is linked to a number of ideas and expressions. I have space to mention only a few here. These and others are elaborated further throughout this book. Two excellent supporting texts on empowerment are Jack (1995) and Kendall (1998). What follows here are some thumbnail sketches of conceptions of empowerment. Hopefully, they will act to sensitise the reader to the richness of the term and help to frame what comes later. The sketches which follow are not mutually exclusive, but overlap and interrelate.

It means what you want it to mean

I wonder if empowerment is:

> *any more than a fancy name for doing a good job as a leader, manager or supervisor, or is an empowerer just an all-round good egg who is always willing to help anyone who needs a bit of support? A concept to make something ordinary sound "academic" and "theoretical", or just plain common sense?... And does it matter what it means*

> *anyway as long as the people who use it know what they mean and how they interpret empowerment in the context of their work?*
>
> (Bell and Harrison, 1998, p.66)

Wallcraft (1994) also reminds us that empowerment, like reflection, has many meanings:

> *For some people empowerment may mean having a place on the management committee or the local joint care planning team. Some people may feel empowered by beginning to write poetry or by setting up a self-help group to reduce their dependence on drugs. For some it means getting a good job, going back to college or making new relationships. For others empowerment means ceasing to try to meet the expectations of society and simply living life in their own way at last... Empowerment is risky, but it is our right as human beings.*
>
> (p.9)

Empowerment, then, can be seen to cover a wide range of activities,

> *... from the power of users to choose what care is provided and how, through involvement and participation in service planning and delivery, to user control of public services.*
>
> (Jack, 1995, p.14)

Empowerment as a good thing:

Throughout much of the literature on empowerment there is an assumption that it is a 'good thing'. Some argue that it is better to be empowered than disempowered. Some say that being empowered is about being more effective, productive, fulfilled and healthier. The claims listed above all relate — to a greater or lesser extent — to this broad conception of empowerment which has been described as a 'myopia of therapeutic good intention' (Jack, 1995).

Empowerment of the individual

When associated with the individual, empowerment is often called 'self-empowerment'. This term is linked to ideas of self-care, self-responsibility, self-determination, and personal control and struggle (Kendall, 1998). It is to do with individuals taking control of their circumstances, achieving their personal desires and goals and trying to enhance the quality of their lives (Adams, 1990).

Collective empowerment

Going beyond individualism, empowerment is often expressed in terms of relationships between individuals, with issues of group or community empowerment. This is often linked with the idea of an empowering partnership (Le May, 1998; Tones, 1993) which may occur, for example, in certain nurse/patient relationships. In relation to community empowerment, Tones (1998) raises the question: 'Is an empowered community merely the sum of those empowered individuals who are members of that community?' (p.189). He goes on to suggest that a 'sense of community' is a central feature of a healthy, empowered community. He refers to the work of McMillan and Chavis (1986) to help him define the characteristics of a sense of community. These are:

- membership — a feeling of belonging
- shared emotional connection — a commitment to be together
- influence — a sense of mattering
- integration and fulfilment of needs — through being a member of the community.

These qualities are worth bearing in mind as we strive to build empowered healthcare teams.

Empowerment as a commodity

Then we have the idea of empowerment as a commodity, bestowed on those without it by those who have it to give. It is a commodity that is given or withheld. If you have it, you are empowered; if not, then you are disempowered. This is a crude and simplistic view, linked to the consumer movement in healthcare in the 1980s and 90s. If empowerment is seen as something bestowed on healthcare workers and their clients/patients by those people who have it to give, rather than as something personally acquired through struggle and negotiation, then it might be better to regard it as just another form of social control or oppression (Ghaye and Ghaye, 1998; Piper and Brown, 1998).

Empowerment as a process

In contrast to this, some hold the view of empowerment as a process where, for instance, individuals or groups transform themselves in some beneficial manner. This usually involves some commitment to a 'cause' or a vision. The process is described in many ways and can involve certain strategies or steps. For example, within this conception we find the idea that empowerment is rather like a 'pass-it-on' process. This concept finds expression thus: 'Nurses themselves must first be empowered in order to be able to empower others' (Latter, 1998, p.24). Another concept is of the 'give-it-away' process. Again, this finds expression in such phrases as: 'We have to relinquish power, our role as expert, and pass control over to others.' This, of course, is potentially threatening for both parties. We can also find evidence of empowerment described as an 'enablement' process. This view asserts that the process is not so much about giving power away, as about creating opportunities which enable and encourage power to be taken. Then there is empowerment as 'a process of becoming' (Keiffer, 1984). Keiffer describes the empowerment process as having four stages. Firstly, there is an exploratory stage where authority and power structures are demystified. It is a kind of reconnaissance stage. Secondly there is an 'era of advancement', where strategies for action are developed. Thirdly comes an 'era of incorporation' in which the barriers to increased self-determination are confronted. Finally we have an 'era of commitment', where new knowledge and skills help to create new realities. In an interesting book by Johnson and Redmond (1998), empowerment is described as an 'art' and the pinnacle of employee involvement. The process whereby an organisation moves away from a hierarchical 'command and control' culture towards one of empowerment, is associated with employee 'profit and pain' and a shift in the power matrix. Empowering workers often involves a change in management style and in the culture of the organisation.

Empowerment as a way of thinking

This has been espoused by McDougall (1997). It serves to remind us that empowerment should not be reduced to a series of techniques or methods. It is more fundamental. We can align this to Dewey's (1933) view of reflection which he described as a whole 'way of being'. How we think affects what we do.

Empowerment as using power

Clearly, 'empowerment' means something different to each of those who hold various different conceptions of power. Discussions about empowerment inevitably involve notions of the related concept of power — what it is, who has and does not have it, who wants it and cannot get it, who has it and does not want it, and who does what with it. Power is a complex and slippery notion. For some it is about sectional interests, territoriality, giving and gaining ground, about domination and dependence. When these are understood in relation to empowerment, it takes us into the area of social justice (Griffiths, 1998). Enhancing justice and becoming more empowered means that we have to understand and alter existing power relations.

Empowerment as developing a voice

Empowerment is also linked to the ways in which people resist, confront and alter the 'structures' which serve to constrain thinking and action in certain healthcare work environments. Empowerment, in this sense, is associated with the critical idea of 'voice'. Voice is the connection between reflection and action. If healthcare workers feel that they are a group upon which power is brought to bear to ensure their compliance and 'domesticity' to prevailing values and routines, then their voice is as one of the oppressed (Ryles, 1999). Challenging this hegemony is about developing a voice and making it heard.

> *This, it can be argued, will be achieved by a commitment to the raising of political consciousness within nurses as a means of not only having them recognise the current nature of their position but also beginning to challenge and change those circumstances.*
>
> (Ryles, 1999, p.605–6)

In this sense, 'voice' is used to enable healthcare professionals to resist becoming colonised or domesticated in the service of the status quo. By implication, then, empowerment is concerned with confronting oppression.

Voice is about communication. Being empowered is not simply a process of 'giving a voice'; it is more complicated than this. Here the ideas of Habermas (1977) are helpful. In essence, Habermas argued that power is often exercised through the manipulation and/or distortion of communication. This means that individuals and groups have a different say in what passes for 'reality', for the shared view, the consensus. He also argued that communication was largely directed, not towards reaching agreement, but rather towards the achievement of ends — the achievement of the ends of those whose interests the communication expresses and reflects. These ends can be achieved through argument, but also through the exercise of power. The power to control agendas, to use knowledge possessed by the privileged few, through authority. This also reflects Lukes' (1974) view about:

> *the way powerful élite groups are able to persuade less powerful groups to hold views or act in ways which are contrary to their own interests.*
>
> (Griffiths, 1998, p.56)

In the context of the rhetoric of *A First Class Service: Quality in the New NHS* (HMSO, 1998) and initiatives such as Clinical Governance, it is critical that we strive to understand whose interests are being served and what power structures underlie this.

Empowerment as a discourse

Elsewhere in Ghaye and Ghaye (1998) I have argued that reflective practices need to be understood as a discourse. The same can be said of empowerment. A discourse can be understood as a set of meanings, statements, stories, and so on which produce a particular version of events. Those who share and support a particular view of things, or a particular version of events, can be regarded as a group or a community. The discourse serves to create an identity for the community; it can create a niche or position for its members in relation to other discourse communities and can link them to, or separate them from, other communities. We cannot become part of a group if we do not understand the language the members use or the reasons why they value or interpret events in the way that they do. So,

> *discourse is about more than language. Discourse is about the interplay between language and social relationships, in which some groups are able to achieve dominance for their interests in the way in which the world is defined and acted upon... Language is a central aspect of discourse through which power is reproduced and communicated.*
>
> (Hugman, 1991)

There are many kinds of discourse. For example, in relation to mental health, Tilley *et al* (1999) refer to the work of Glenister and Tilley (1996), who describe a:

> *dominant 'medical' discourse characterising mental illness, for example schizophrenia, as a long-term disabling illness,*
>
> *a 'social disablement' discourse locating the primary obstacles to social integration in the environment rather than the person,*
>
> *a 'human rights' discourse focusing on the 'degrading' aspects of mental health care provision and relating social integration to social justice issues,*
>
> *a 'consumerist' discourse reframing the patient or client as a user of services.*
>
> (pp.54–5)

There are, of course, many other discourses which are of significance and enlighten healthcare work. For example, from the field of feminist studies there is a growing discourse on the empowerment of women. In all of these discourses there is a need to understand the complex social, historical and political influences which serve to constrain or liberate people and shape their lives. Tilley *et al* (1999) ask us to be cautious and not unwittingly to 'pitch in with the dominant discourses' (p.58). Reflective practices help us to make reasoned decisions about which discourses we value and use. These practices can reveal to us which discourses — and therefore groups — are being privileged and which peripheralised.

Empowerment as a personal reality

I would like to offer a personal view of empowerment which is derived from my interactions with a variety of professionals in health and education, and from my understandings of the literature. I suggest that *empowerment is about individuals and groups coming to know, express and critically analyse their own realities and having the commitment, will and power to act to transform these realities to enhance personal and collective well-being, security, satisfaction, capability and working conditions.*

This view raises such questions as: Whose reality? Whose fantasy? What power? and Will people have to act in this way? I shall return to this conception of empowerment and substantiate it further in the following sections of this chapter.

Where are some of the roots of empowerment? Realities from afar

I have already suggested that there is a view of empowerment which is associated with the struggle of oppressed individuals and groups for greater dignity and self-determination. This struggle is about becoming more fully ourselves; more valued, respected and fulfilled. Notions of perceived injustice or oppression are almost always linked with the idea of empowerment. If empowerment, in one sense, is about such people as healthcare workers and patients taking action to gain more control over their own lives (Grace, 1991), then we have to decide, for example, whether this is a desirable moral and ethical principle; a personal, professional and/or political process. This view of personal empowerment, of people trying to take more control of themselves and changing their lives for the better (Schafer, 1996), is wonderfully illustrated in the work of Friere (1972, 1974, 1985, 1994). Reading his work helps us, in a very vivid way, to understand the roots of some of our current thinking about empowerment. You may also find his writing inspiring and energising.

A Brazilian man, Paulo Friere is known worldwide as an educator. Friere's educational theory centres upon the concept of 'progressive education'. This is linked to ideas about education as political practice; to ideas about oppression, competence, utopias and empowerment. His work addresses the impossibility of neutral practice and the virtues, such as humility, tolerance and love, which should shape the practices of the educator.

During a visit to London in 1993, Friere's wife spoke of her husband's work, begun with the illiterate population in NE Brazil:

> *Paulo Friere has become a political-pedagogue of the oppressed, of all those who wish to re-invent, from the furnace of colonialism, a just and non-eternally dependent society; of all those so-called minorities (women, blacks, homosexuals, migrants, etc) who need and are willing to participate actively and not marginally, precisely because they have been excluded from the actions of their country and their community; of all those who, suffering from class discrimination, hunger, lack of housing and schools are unable to name the world because society, closed in its privileges, does not permit them to have; to be; to wish; to know. We wish those people, no matter how they are named — excluded, oppressed or proscribed — to have, to*

> *be, to wish, to be able to and to know, and therefore to name the world.*
>
> (de Figueiredo-Cowen and Gastaldo, 1995, p.27)

Reflective practices which seek to empower practitioners owe much to the work and inspiration of Friere, to the practice and experience of 'conscientisation' and the development of 'authentic dialogues' in Latin America. The terms 'conscientisation' and 'dialogue' are central to Friere's thinking and work. Conscientisation:

> *is a process of developing consciousness, but a consciousness that is understood to have the power to transform reality.*
>
> (Taylor, 1993, p.52)

For Friere, reality is a social construction. This means that we build meanings and construct identities for ourselves within a cultural, historical and political context. We develop a personal reality which is something we perceive, claim to know and believe. It is a reality which we experience and put together ourselves. Personal realities all differ. We all see things differently.

> *Personal realities are... complex, diverse and dynamic. We speak then of a world of multiple realities, in which each of us constructs our own and has our own way of constructing what we perceive.*
>
> (Chambers, 1997, p.57)

In any discussion about reality, questions of the following kind must be addressed: What reality? Whose reality? and Whose reality counts? In healthcare, just as there are dominant dialogues (or discourses), for example a medical discourse, so too there are dominant realities which are often top-down, centre-periphery-transferred realities. Sometimes these realities override locally known and owned realities. Sometimes they do not fit and are therefore rejected or become grounds for discontent. The challenging question is: Whose reality constitutes the 'real' and therefore the basis for action?

For Friere, dialogue is a process by and through which we transform and recreate the world. Conscientisation, as a process of becoming more aware of the oppressor and of understanding the means by which oppression is sustained, is fostered by dialogue. It is a means of transforming the oppressed into the liberated. Dialogue is therefore essential for a 'liberating education'. It is a process of coming to know. It is a way of 'revealing a reality' to ourselves and actually 'transforming that reality'. It is, therefore, a potentially creative and liberating process. For Friere,

> *dialogue is loving, humble, hopeful, trusting and critical... more simply put... without dialogue one cannot be human.*
>
> (Taylor, 1993, p.62)

In his work, Friere reminds us that thinking and dialogue should not be done alone. They move us from the 'I' to the 'we'. There should be a co-participation in the process of initiating and sustaining meaningful and authentic dialogue. If we are deprived of dialogue, we are oppressed. Dialogue is the practice of liberation. It involves critical thinking about the mutually interactive way individuals and society inform and transform each other. In healthcare we have to make important choices between seeing dialogues, of one form or another, as instruments of domination or liberation.

All this is very heady stuff, but it is not 'out there', abstract and irrelevant to the everyday practices of healthcare workers. How can the essence of Frierian work, which argues that exploited, marginalised, vulnerable, disaffected and disempowered people can and should be enabled to express and analyse their own realities and go on to plan and act in ways that transform them, be anything other than central and fundamental to that which we describe as 'caring work'? However, much still needs to be done to join up Frierian thinking and caring work. Much more needs to be done to move from revealing realities to transforming them. This will involve a big shift for many in their understandings of the nature and purposes of reflective practices. Such a shift will reveal the more political and militant face of reflection. Some Frierian principles and processes are surfacing in healthcare. For example, in the excellent text by Johns and Freshwater (1998) we can detect some attempt at linkage being made. The title of the book is *Transforming Nursing through Reflective Practice*. Although there are only two references to the work of Friere in the book, they are significant ones. The first refers to nurses who perceived themselves as an oppressed group within a system which denied them access to higher degrees in the field of nursing (Lumby, 1998). The second appears in a discussion of reflection and the development of 'expert' nursing knowledge. Reflection is described as a liberating and empowering process, catalysed by critical thinking and consciousness (Glaze, 1998).

> *This ability to become critically conscious is far removed from simply examining an event to see what should be*

done differently. There is an implicit political dimension, linked to critical awareness, which enables assumptions inherent in ideologies to be challenged.

(Johns and Freshwater, 1998, p.152)

How far does empowerment involve reversals in power?

Thus far I have briefly sketched out some of the ways in which empowerment has been described and experienced. I am coming to a point in the discussion where I believe that it is appropriate to suggest again that *empowerment is about individuals and groups coming to know, express and critically analyse their own realities as well as having the commitment, will and power to act to transform these realities to enhance personal and collective well-being, security, satisfaction, capability and working conditions*.

This view raises the questions: What power? and Will people have to act in this way? In this view of empowerment, I am espousing the primacy and power of the individual and the group. It is a view that appreciates the power of personal and collective choice. It is a view that requires certain reversals in power. It acknowledges that power is 'positioned' historically, socially, politically and also economically.

So, what do we mean when we use the term 'power'? Just like 'empowerment' and 'reflection', 'power' is understood and used in many ways. It is used by us explicitly, and also alluded to in our daily work in relation to a myriad of things — for example, in relation to getting things done, effective leadership, overcoming resistance, managing change, handling conflict, giving rewards, making people feel good or depressed, communicating effectively, team building and working collaboratively. Then, of course, there are well-used expressions such as 'the powerful', 'the powerless', 'knowledge is power' (Smith, 1996) and 'power dressing'. We then also have power being used, more or less synonymously, with such words as 'manipulation', 'force', 'coercion' and 'imposition'. But we should remember that exercising power is not a one-way process. For example, when a healthcare group is formed, some members may exercise power by exclusion: some people are in; others are out. The excluded may also exercise power by usurping, challenging or sabotaging the composition and work of the group.

There are also gendered views of power. For example, in Benner (1984), where the author is discussing 'excellence and power in clinical nursing practice', we find:

> *Excellence requires commitment and involvement, but it also requires power. Since caring is central to nursing, then power without excellence is an anathema. I am concerned when I hear nurses say that the very qualities essential to their caring role are the source of their powerlessness in the male-dominated hospital hierarchy. Such a statement disparages feminine qualities and elevates a masculine view of power, one that emphasises competitiveness, domination and control. But to define power or nursing exclusively in traditional masculine or feminine terms is a mistake. The disparagement of feminine perspectives on power is based upon the misguided assumption that feminine values have kept women and nursing subservient, rather than recognising that society's devaluing of and discrimination against women are the sources of the problem.*
>
> (pp.207–8)

Griffiths (1998) and Hugman (1991) provide some very helpful frameworks for us to begin to understand the term, 'power'. The ways in which power is understood and exercised, and the ways it impacts on individuals and groups are complex. There is space here only to raise some general and relatively more understandable ideas. Lukes (1974) emphasises the social nature of power and alerts us to a distinction between 'power over' and 'power to act'. These two phrases identify two broad approaches which we can use to aid understanding of power. The first is a view of power as an aspect of social relationships. The second is power as an element of social action. Hugman (1991) suggests that:

> *If power is not an isolated element of social life, but one which interweaves occupational and organisational structures with the actions of professionals, individually and collectively, then it must be examined in terms of the contexts within which the caring professions are structured and operate.*
>
> (Ibid, p.38)

He goes on further, suggesting that:

> *... the caring professions cannot be understood without reference to issues of hierarchy, occupation, the clientele, race and gender, which are not isolated from each other in the lived historical world.*
>
> (Ibid, p.50)

I shall briefly mention three things here. Firstly, power in relation to the notion of hierarchy. Qualifications and experience create levels, for example as reflected in grades, within healthcare. Seniority can be seen as power and authority over junior staff. Seniority confers power and is a taken-for-granted fact of life for many. When all those in the occupational hierarchy see it this way and do not question it, the power structure is secure and remains in tact.

Secondly, power in relation to the notion of occupation. In occupations such as nursing and in the many professions allied to medicine, for example, the occupation represents a power structure within itself. But potent power relationships also exist between occupations. The clearest example of this is the way the medical profession has historically exercised power over nursing and the remedial therapies. In relation to nursing, for example, and a duty of care, the development of a self-confident profession can be seen to be held back by a deep anti-intellectual prejudice attached to women's work in general and to the gendering of skill more particularly. This is where discussions about power get us into deep issues to do with the intellectual and social subordination of those discharging caring work. It invites us to understand the links between power, authority, knowledge production and practice.

Thirdly, we need to understand power as it expresses itself within a context. This reminds us of the interconnectedness of the aspects of power mentioned here. The interconnectedness between social relationships (those involved), social action (what is or is not happening) and the context in which it is embedded. Context has historical, social, political, economic (resource), as well as spatial dimensions. For example, 'connecting' with a patient at a bedside can be understood like this and in relation to the earlier issues of hierarchy, occupation, social class, gender, race, and so on. The understanding of power in a context is beautifully described by Benner (1984). She argues that nurses do have power, though they exert their power from a position of low status in the hierarchy. In examining nursing practice, she describes six 'qualities of power' and names them: transformative power, integrative caring, advocacy, healing power, participative/affirmative power and problem solving.

So, how far can we argue that empowerment involves some reversals in power? I can only briefly sketch in some of the main ideas here (for more detail, see Ghaye and Lillyman, 2000). I have presented a view of empowerment as one which describes the way individuals and groups come to know, express and critically analyse their own realities. I have also argued that there are multiple realities which are socially constructed. There are also dominant realities which can stifle, oppress and silence. These realities belong to élite and powerful individuals and groups who impose their reality on others. We can see power as an asset and a means of getting things done. We can also view 'power as a disability' (Chambers, 1997). It is held by those who cannot easily be contradicted or corrected. It is a case of 'their word goes'. By imposing their realities and denying those of others, it is often difficult for the 'powerful' to learn.

By implication, 'reversals in power' also involve 'reversals in reality'. We can attempt to achieve this by shifts in orientation (the way we see our caring work), in relationships (how we work with each other) and in activity (what we do). These are not discrete categories, as the following illustrates. For example, I suggest that becoming empowered requires certain reversals in power which involve at least:

- **Developing a more reflective posture**
  This requires healthcare professionals to fully embrace both the principles and practices of reflection. Learning and constructing meaningful realities is then about active reflection and reflective action. It is about becoming more aware of how we learn; how this affects what we think, feel and do and how reflection reveals to us how we construct our own reality and distort the realities of others.
- **Questioning transfers of reality**
  This involves questioning top-down, outside-in and centre-periphery transfers of healthcare policy and practices. It is questioning such 'truths' as: 'If it is good for them, it must be good for this group' and 'If it works here, then it must work over there, too!'and 'If we understand it to mean this, then they will understand it to mean the same thing.' Simple transfers of reality can misfit with local needs, wants and values.
- **Challenging those who dominate from a distance**
  This is about listening to and acknowledging the realities of the individual, the particular, the 'grounded' and the local, and not just the realities of senior managers, executives and those in the

research 'academy'. This links with the Frierian notions I mentioned earlier of conscientisation and authentic dialogues.

- **Reversals in sources of commitment**
The less power people have in shaping and controlling their professional lives, the less commitment they will have. When senior managers single-handedly define the working conditions and expectations of healthcare professionals, all that employees do is what is expected of them. When tasks, behaviours and performance are defined by 'others' and come from 'elsewhere', and when the value of what we do is defined by outsiders, empowerment, in the way I have described it in this chapter, will not be an authentically-lived experience. Empowerment is about commitments that come from within.
- **Valuing our own practical knowledge and not just the knowledge of others**
One of the most divisive, inhibiting, oppressive and pervasive beliefs in much of healthcare is that the only knowledge worth having and knowing is that which is 'scientific' and propositional in kind. This is knowledge which is derived from randomised control trials, from large samples, and which uses a hypothetico-deductive approach. It is knowledge which claims to be generalisable and universally 'true'. It also carries with it the spurious label of being 'objective' knowledge. It carries with it a sense of 'certainty'. Whilst not denying the value of knowledge of this kind for certain purposes, I do believe that empowerment requires a significant reversal in our usual answer to the question: 'So what knowledge is worth knowing?' Just as reality is ambiguous and uncertain, so too is knowledge. Really worthwhile knowledge can be generated in many ways. We might expect empowered healthcare workers to value and celebrate knowledge which is constructed from the descriptions and explanations they give of their own local practice (Whitehead, 1993).
- **By embracing uncertainty and contradiction rather than a standardised, controlled and predictable world**
In healthcare, change is continuous. Therefore, realities are multiple and in constant flux. The world has had to adapt itself to a permanence of transitions. We have to work safely and accountably at the edge of chaos (Gleick, 1988; Ghaye, 1996). Almost everything needs to be permanently provisional. Empowerment enables us to reverse much of our normal thinking about 'how the world is', 'appears to be' and 'should be'.

Empowerment and the emperor's new clothes

I began this chapter by retelling the story of the emperor's new clothes. The narrative illuminates many of the golden threads I have used to weave a pattern in words which might serve to clarify the nature of empowerment and how it can be known, experienced and analysed through reflective practices. Centrally, it has been about understanding empowerment through a reflection upon views of power and reality. The ministers, courtiers, chamberlains and all those who cheered on the procession, reflect the disempowered in the emperor's kingdom. Fear of losing their jobs and fear of being seen as fools makes them the oppressed in the emperor's kingdom. There are contradictions between what they really see and know and what they say and do. The pressures and expectations which bear down on them trap, enslave and imprison them. Their cheering and shouting serves only to sustain a false and alien reality. It is not their reality, but someone else's. The presence of the small boy in the story is hugely symbolic. He is able to question what is before him. The ability to ask a question serves to break the mould. It is liberating. We have learnt in this chapter that some are more able to ask questions than others; some are more able to challenge the status quo; some are more able to ask:

- Whose values matter?
- Whose knowledge counts?
- Whose action?
- Whose interests are being served?
- Whose learning?
- Whose reality?
- Whose empowerment?

References

Adams R (1990) *Self-help, Social work and Empowerment.* Macmillan, Basingstoke

Bell J, Harrison B (1998) *Leading People: Learning from People.* Open University Press, Milton Keynes

Benner P (1984) *From Novice to Expert: Excellence and Power in Clinical Nursing Practice.* Addison-Wesley, California

Chambers R (1997) *Whose Reality Counts? Putting the First Last.* Intermediate Technology Publication, London de Figueiredo-Cowen M, Gastaldo D (1995) *Paulo Friere at the Institute.* Institute of Education, University of London, London

Department of Health (1998) *A First Class Service: Quality in the New NHS.* HMSO, London

Dewey J (1933) *How we think.* Henry Regnery, Chicago

Friere P (1972) *Pedagogy of the Oppressed.* Sheed and Ward, London

Friere P (1974) *Education for Critical Consciousness.* Sheed and Ward, London

Friere P (1985) *The Politics of Education: culture, power and liberation.* Bergin and Garvey, South Hadley, Mass.

Friere P (1994) *Pedagogy of Hope.* Continuum, New York

Ghaye T (1996) Critical Reflective Practice: Towards the big simplicity. In: Ghaye T, ed (1996) *Reflection and Action for Healthcare Professionals: A Reader*. Pentaxion Press, Newcastle-Upon-Tyne

Ghaye T *et al* (1996) *Theory-Practice Relationships: Reconstructing Practice.* Pentaxion Press, Newcastle-Upon-Tyne

Ghaye T, Ghaye K (1998) T*eaching and Learning through Critical Reflective Practice.* David Fulton, London

Ghaye T, Lillyman S (2000) *Reflection: Principles and Practice for Healthcare Professionals.* Quay Books, Mark Allen Publishing Ltd, Salisbury

Glaze J (1998) Reflection and Expert Nursing Knowledge. In: Johns C, Freshwater D, eds (1998) *Transforming Nursing through Reflective Practice.* Blackwell Science, Oxford

Gleick J (1988) *Chaos: Making a New Science.* Sphere Books, Penguin Group, London

Glenister D, Tilley S (1996) Discourse, social exclusion and empowerment. *J Psychiatr Mental Health Nurs* **3** (1): 3–5

Grace V (1991) The marketing of empowerment and the construction of the health consumer; a critique of health promotion. *Int J Health Stud* **21** (2): 329–43

Griffiths M (1998) *Educational Research for Social Justice: getting off the fence.* Open University Press, Milton Keynes

Habermas J (1974) *Theory and Practice.* Heinemann, London

Habermas J (1977) Hannah Arendt's communications concept of power. *Soc Res* **44** (1): 3–24

Hugman R (1991) *Power in Caring Professions.* Macmillan Press, Basingstoke

Jack R ed (1995) *Empowerment in Community Care.* Chapman and Hall, London

James C, Clarke B (1994) Reflective Practice in Nursing Issues and Implications for Nurse Education. *Nurse Educ Today* **14**: 8–90

Johns C, Freshwater D, eds (1998) *Transforming Nursing through Reflective Practice.* Blackwell Science, Oxford

Johnson R, Redmond D (1998) *The Art of Empowerment.* Pitman Publishing, London

Keiffer C (1984) Citizen Empowerment: a developmental perspective. *Prevention in Human Services* **3**: 9–36

Kendall S (1998) *Health and Empowerment: Research and Practice.* Arnold, London

Knowles M (1970) *The Modern Practice of Adult Education: pedagogy to andragogy.* Cambridge Book Company, Cambridge

Kolb D (1984) *Experiential Learning: experience as a source of learning and development.* Prentice Hall, New Jersey

Latter S (1998) Health promotion in the acute setting; the case for empowering nurses. In: Kendall S (1998) *Health and Empowerment: Research and Practice.* Arnold, London

Le May A (1998) Communication Skills. In: Redfern S, Ross F, eds *Nursing Elderly People.* Harcourt Brace, Edinburgh

Lukes S (1974) *Power: A radical view.* Macmillan, London

Lumby J (1998) Transforming Nursing through Reflective Practice. In: Johns C, Freshwater D, eds (1998) *Transforming Nursing through Reflective Practice.* Blackwell Science, Oxford

McDougall L (1997) Patient Empowerment: fact or fiction? *Ment Health Nurs* **17**: 4–5

McMillan D, Chavis D (1986) Sense of Community: a definition and theory. *J Community Psychol* **14**: 6–23

McSherry R, Haddock J (1999) Evidence-based health care: its place within clinical governance. *Br J Nurs* **8** (2): 113–7

McTaggart R (1994) Participatory Action Research. *Educational Action Res J* **2** (3): 313–37

Mezirow J (1981) A Critical Theory of Adult Learning and Adult Education. *Adult Educ* **32** (1): 3–24

Piper S, Brown P (1998) Psychology as a theoretical foundation for health education in nursing; empowerment or social control? *Nurse Educ Today* **18**: 637–41

Powell J (1989) The reflective practitioner in nursing. *J Adv Nurs* **14**: 824–32

Rushton B (1999) Pause for Thought. *Mental Health Care* **2** (8): 277–9

Ryles S (1999) A concept analysis of empowerment: its relationship to mental health nursing. *J Adv Nurs* **29** (3): 600–7

Schafer T (1996) Empowering Service Users: the myth, the reality and the hope. *J Psychiatr Mental Health Nurs* **3**: 391–4

Schon D (1983) *The Reflective Practitioner.* Basic Books Inc., New York

Smith J (1996) *Empowering People.* Kogan Page, London

Taylor P (1993) *The Texts of Paulo Friere.* Open University Press, Milton Keynes

Tilley S, Pollock L, Tait L (1999) Discourses on Empowerment. *J Psychiatr Mental Health Nurs* **6**: 53–60

Tones K (1993) The Theory of Health Promotion: implications for nursing. In: Wilson-Barnett J, Macleod C, eds (1993) *Research in Health Promotion and Nursing.* Macmillan, Basingstoke

Tones K (1998) Empowerment for Health: the challenge. In: Kendall S (1998) *Health and Empowerment: Research and Practice.* Arnold, London

Wallcraft J (1994) Empowering Empowerment: Professionals and self-advocacy projects. *Mental Health Nurs* **14** (2): 6–9

Whitehead J (1993) *The Growth of Educational Knowledge: Creating your own living educational theories.* Hyde Publications, Bournmouth

6

Power: Its holders and effects on nursing

Dave Gillespie

Many nurses may think that power is not a particularly important or relevant issue when it comes to their daily practice. Some may think otherwise. They are almost certain to feel that the issue of disempowerment is very relevant. For most nurses — and I dare say individuals from other health and educational disciplines — power is something they feel coming from around them, exerting its influence upon them and their practice, even if for the majority of the time they are far too busy to think about it. Perhaps an appropriate synonym would be 'pressure' or perhaps 'stress'. Most nurses would see this pressure as coming from two main sources — managers and doctors.

Many nurses feel that managers make practitioners' lives very difficult, and that the manager who is empowering is a very rare phenomenon. The aims of management in many areas of healthcare organisations are to ensure that policy is implemented in every area; that nurses do their job; that the needs of every patient are met, often in situations where wards and community teams are overstretched, under-resourced and have too few staff. As for doctors, many nurses may see them as simply awesome in their possession of power. Nurses may feel totally intimidated and experience a certain 'fear' of the consultant or consultants they work with. For many, ward rounds have been a traditional nightmare. The opinions of the consultant can override any considerations nurses may have — arguably, nurses merely provide information and woe betide them if they are wrong! Nurse educators also play an important role. From their days of training through to their subsequent time as registered nurses and taking any courses they may follow, many nurses see their teachers as being highly influential.

However, nurses themselves are not individuals totally without power. By their being closest to the patients, they have a degree — and some might say a large degree — of power. In many areas of nursing, perhaps with the exception of psychiatry, the patient will, on most occasions, do what the nurse asks them to do.

The power which is exerted on the nurse, the power which she uses, and the disempowerment she experiences are issues which require some investigation.

So, what of power? What do we mean by this word? Well, in this instance, I am referring to power in a sociological sense, that is, looking at how it operates between people. I feel it is important to state that I am a practising psychiatric nurse. Hence, some of my ideas may appear to focus in the direction of psychiatry. Having said this, I feel that much of what I intend to discuss will be relevant to all nurses in all specialities, as well as to others from further afield. Farmer (1993) states that 'power is one of the most evocative words in the English language'. Hokanson Hawks (1991) conducted an inquiry into what power might be. She provided a brief history of the word, initially referring back to the Latin, Middle English and Anglo-French periods. She then identified a group of synonyms: 'influence, clout, prestige, control, authority, dominance, efficacy, command and force' (Hokanson Hawks, 1991, p.754). Later on in her discussion she makes an important discovery: that she prefers to see power as having a 'power to' orientation rather than a 'power over' one.

Gilbert (1995) suggests that power fits within two broad areas. The first is the humanistic model, which relies largely upon the idea that power belongs to each individual and can be expanded through personal growth. The second takes the position that power is more of a communal phenomenon in which power is produced with greater effect where people work together — this is the notion of synergy.

What we are beginning to see, here, is the diversity of ways of looking at the concept of power — different authors have various perceptions of power. If we examine Hokanson Hawks' list of synonyms, we see that the vast majority of them give power a perspective of superiority. Power, in such cases, is about having control, authority, dominance; it is about being able to implement the things you want, whether or not other people agree with you. It is holding a position of being able to decide and put into practice exactly what you wish to. This is very different from the 'power to' concept which is about having power to do things on a personal basis.

Gilbert's perspective on power is slightly different. Initially, he looks at personal power; the power of the individual. He considers, through the humanistic model, the belief that personal power can be enhanced and developed; that individuals can become whatever they want to become. He also makes reference to the important notion that the fact of people working closely together will result in each individual eventually having more power. Here, then, we are looking at the power of the person but there are, of course, other factors which affect individuals and so need to be considered. Individuals have (or may have) a certain degree of power, but they operate within a wider societal group. Within this group there are other people, or groups of people, who have more or less power than they do. Here, then, we begin to see the conceptualisation of power becoming broader — we now see power as an interpersonal phenomenon.

Interpersonal power is obviously something of which nurses and many others will have much experience. Indeed, this is probably true of everyone. We all experience moments with others when we feel in a position of dominance, or equality, or inferiority. Hewison (1995) takes a look at interpersonal power, examining nurses' power in their interactions with patients. He refers to French and Raven (1959) who suggested that interpersonal power is:

> *characterized by 'give and take' in interactions and is generally through one party having a 'base', be it information, reward or coercion, which constitutes their power over others.*

Here, power is seen as knowing something which someone else doesn't, for example, which can then be used to influence situations to the benefit of the information holder.

Hewison also recognises that, traditionally, nursing has been viewed as possessing relatively little power within the healthcare service. We are now going beyond the issue of the interpersonal and into the relative positions of groups of workers who have, or do not have, the power to affect the organisation of healthcare. In the majority of developed countries, the healthcare organisation is monumental. There are many individuals and groups who directly affect the way it is run. In Britain there is the government, the Secretary of State for Health, and the Department of Health, all of whom interact with senior members of the medical profession and senior health service management. The decisions which these people make trickle down through the system and directly affect the way the service runs. Perhaps unfortunately, it would appear that nurses have very little influence at this level. Indeed, there is even legislation which governs the practice of nursing (Pyne, 1994). There have been calls for nurses to become more political, to begin to be involved in macro-level decision making (Taylor, 1995), and it would certainly seem odd that the group of workers which is overwhelmingly the largest in healthcare provision should have so little political influence.

So now we have touched upon the various areas where power operates — from the personal to the governmental. Let us, for the time being, return to the local — to the hospital and take a more in-depth look at power and how it operates there. Firstly, we can observe one of the local power holders, the management, and the impact which managers have on the practice of nurses. In their study, Brewer and Lok (1995) examine managers, referring in the background to their research to the issue of 'organisational commitment'. They see organisational commitment as being:

> *... linked to the employee's acceptance of a managerial strategy based on plans, policies and processes, for structuring accountability and decision-making and for designing work and the employment contract.*
>
> (Brewer and Lok, 1995, p.790)

They go on to discuss the variety of issues related to the notion of the 'committed worker'. Committed workers have, they suggest,

> *a desire to remain employed, a willingness to invest efforts in their jobs, regular attendance at work and an attempt to balance managerial and their own interests. Committed employees are more productive, show more initiative, and help to create a more effective work organisation.*
>
> (Brewer and Lok, 1995, p.790)

Here, then, is the ideal relationship between an employer and employees who feel so content with the way their organisation is run that they show complete commitment. I wonder how many nurses feel this way. To produce and maintain such a contented workforce would require exceptional management. Employees would expect recognition, rewards for efforts, good working conditions, potential for promotion, access to further training, a supportive management position — in fact a whole range of things. Of course, in reality, this is often not the case and, further than this, management may wish to implement strategies or policies with which the employee simply does not agree. Indeed, in modern healthcare there seems to be something of a difference between the aims of nurses and those of their managers, some feeling that they share 'a common occupation in name only' (Porter, 1992, p.721).

Porter highlights a number of other discrepancies. He feels that financial reward increases with 'distance from the bedside' (Porter, 1992, p.721), and stresses that the introduction of generic managers (rather than managers with a nursing background) has caused 'despair in the minds of many nurses' (Porter, 1992, p.722). With the emphasis for managers so much on finance and efficiency, and the emphasis for nurses still so much on patient care, it could be said that there is something of a power struggle developing.

With the governmental financing of health having undergone some radical changes during the eighties and nineties, this struggle has placed both managers and nurses under undoubted pressures. Managers are expected to improve efficiency and run their service on a smaller budget, while, over the years, nurses have seen a gradual decrease in the resources — both human and otherwise — available to them. This has made the nurse's job more difficult and more taxing. But what have nurses, or nursing organisations, done about this? It could be said, 'very little'. Nurses, as indeed the case may always have been, take on the elements of an oppressed group (Farmer, 1993). However, nurse management may not have the same problem. Jacono and Jacono (1994) refer to many papers which portray management as a shining example of trustworthiness and the performers of good deeds. Further, Brewer and Lok (1995), found that the nurses in their study held their nurse unit managers in a positive light and, as a result, demonstrated high work commitment. While certainly acknowledging these findings, there is also evident a considerable mistrust of senior management and administration. The comments of nurses about senior management during interview are, in fact, rather scathing. Generally, it could be said that nurses have something of a fatalistic acceptance of their position, feeling that nothing can be done to influence management decisions so they get on with the job as best they can. In fact, this seems representative of the nurses' attitudes when it comes to many things. There may be much irritating them, bringing them down, but nevertheless they get on with their job. Thus nurses and their managers seem to have different goals in terms of their work and there are also distinct differences in the levels of the power which they hold. Managers implement policy and nurses follow it.

What of the medical profession — a further element of power confronting the nurse? Doctors are recognised in society as being a truly professional body. They enjoy the trust and faith of the majority of people. This relationship has been, largely, historically developed. Doctors are viewed by some as following the archetypal profession (Dingwall and Lewis, 1983) and, as a result, they enjoy certain benefits. They have the ability to self-regulate, hence the existence of the General Medical Council and the British Medical Association. They have a very distinct body of knowledge which is particular to them. Doctors are truly autonomous. However, their service is for the good of the patients whom they serve. Historically, nurses, have always been viewed as the support of the medical service; they carry out the doctors' instructions. At the time when the relationship between doctors and nurses was established, it reflected the way in which society was structured. Most — if not all — doctors were male: the strong, reliable ones; the decision-makers. During the Nightingale era, all nurses were female because they, like many mothers (and few fathers), performed the traditionally female roles of caring and nurturing. Of course, this inevitably brought about an imbalance of power in the relationship, with doctors in the superior position, whilst nurses were perceived to be the inferior partners. Here, it appears, was a further example of oppression representing the socialisation of men and women. This is an arrangement which is still reflected today and is referenced by many feminist writers. Sweet and Norman (1995) discuss the relationship between doctors and nurses in modern times, highlighting the issue of problems between the two occupations. They make reference to the issues of patriarchy and oppression within gender relationships between doctors and nurses. The presence of men in nursing appears to be a problem which doctors would much rather not have to put up with. Men in nursing are perceived as being far more assertive than their female counterparts and, unfortunately for women, climb the promotion ladder of hospitals much quicker. Sweet and Norman (1995) make further reference to some very interesting observations of doctors and nurses, including, amongst others that:

- nurses may carry out instructions from doctors which are very dangerous for patients
- relationships between nurses and senior doctors (that is, consultants) are far worse than relationships between nurses and junior doctors
- in certain circumstances, doctors rely on the knowledge and experience of senior nurses.

The authors also consider the issue of nurses developing more power in their relationship with doctors as a possible reflection of the feminist movement's work in empowering women generally.

May (1995) studies early developments in the two occupations and notes that, from very early on, medicine began to follow scientific principles in its work and that much medical research was conducted in universities. This is a move which nursing did not follow — one possible explanation for the widely-held view that doctors have a stronger body of knowledge than nurses, and a plausible rationale for their greater power and recognition as a profession. Scientific reductionism — a method which is objective and value free, providing explanations for and control of natural phenomena — has been the dominant scientific paradigm for many years. More recently, however, it has come under threat from the alternative ways of pursuing scientific inquiry, that is, the more qualitative approaches.

Nursing theory, as it has developed, began by following a 'hard' scientific methodology in order to be taken seriously as a new science. Today, nursing knowledge is generated in a whole variety of ways, using both quantitative and qualitative approaches. Nursing science is considered by many to be a means by which nursing may pursue its full recognition as a profession (Adams, 1991) and, perhaps, gain increased power. Some feel that the pursuit of professional recognition is not appropriate for nursing. Professionals are seen by some as performing not only in the interests of others but in their own interests. In addition, becoming a qualified member of a profession such as medicine, carries the 'advantage' that only these certain people can do this especially coveted job. It is, apparently, a way of reassuring the public that only its qualified members can conduct practice. It is also a means of controlling rival occupational groups such as, in this case, nurses (Cook, 1992). Indeed, the professionalism of doctors has come in for much criticism from certain writers. Friedson, in Hart (1985), suggests that:

> *The drive to control and dominate the sphere of health and sickness is found in professional ambition itself and the selfless ideology of community service is little more than a means to this end.*
>
> (p.98)

Here, then, we find a position where doctors are not seen as selfless givers to society. Rather, the perception is of a strategy by doctors for concealing their real ambition which is to promote themselves in terms of class and remuneration. Perhaps this would not be an appropriate goal for nursing. In addition to Friedson, there are other authors, such as Illich (1981) and Wilding (1982), who have made similar criticism of the medical profession.

As I mentioned earlier, another body exerting a substantial amount of influence and power upon nurses is the educational establishment or 'academy'. There is considerable debate going on within education. The production of nurses who can bring about a deconstruction of the oppressive forces which currently dominate their practice, appears to be the goal of many educational theorists. However, there seems to be a level of disagreement amongst these theorists as to the best way to achieve this goal. Within nurse education — and indeed education generally — one of the main areas of conflict arises between two different educational approaches: andragogy and pedagogy. Let me explain — and this may help to answer a number of questions which nurses have had regarding their education and training.

Balsamo and Martin (1995) provide a definition of andragogy. Andragogy is seen as:

> *essentially an attempt to encourage educational self-development by conferring on the adult student primary responsibility for the pace and direction of learning.*
>
> (Balsamo and Martin, 1995, p.427)

The authors also provide the following explanation of pedagogy:

> *... the pace and direction of learning are largely controlled by the teacher, whose authority determines what is relevant and significant.*
>
> (Balsamo and Martin, 1995, p.427)

Many nurses I know have not understood these aspects of their training, particularly recent training. They have generally expected to receive the educational style which they received at school — with a pedagogical emphasis. In fact, nurse education was based on the pedagogical approach for many years. The andragogical style has come as a bit of a surprise. There have, however, been problems associated with using this approach to nurse education. Andragogy appears to have a humanistic basis, including the ideas of personal growth and development, of self-awareness and, where possible, of self-actualisation. Purdy (1997) draws attention to various problems associated with this approach. He sees the institutionalisation of learning — nurse education having its base in colleges and universities — as stifling the possibility for nurses to develop personal power and independence. What the humanistic model seems to ignore is the fact that nursing education and practice take place in powerful institutions which restrict, and sometimes even strangle, human agency. Clare (1993) describes health and educational institutions as ‘hegemonic’, defining ‘hegemony’ as:

> *the ability of a dominant class or culture to exercise social and political control, and to legitimate that control, through influencing the consciousness of people to accept its world-view as common sense.*
>
> (Clare, 1993, p.1034)

Whilst nurses may be victims of this institutional hegemony, nurse lecturers themselves have raised their own concerns about the effect institutional hegemony has upon their own practice, and hence on their education of nurses (Gordon and Wimpenny, 1996). Purdy points out that 'liberation and empowerment are social not individual processes' (Purdy, 1997, p.195). Thus, educational theorists have come to identify significant problems with one approach to nurse training. Once again, I refer to Balsamo and Martin (1995) who identify something of a problem with the andragogical approach. Their concern is related to the notions of agency and structure; 'agency' being the ability of an individual to make their own choices free of outside influence, and 'structure' being the world which surrounds them with its possibility of disrupting personal choices. In relation to this concern, the authors take a look at sociology as part of nurse education. They consider the idea of creating an emancipated nurse — one of the aims of Project 2000 — as problematic when this particular trap (that is, how a nurse acts as a free agent within structures which restrict her actions) has not been resolved. This approach, as they state:

> *... promulgates a view of the social world in which frozen subjectivity is enmeshed in a web of deterministic structures.*
>
> (Balsamo and Martin, 1995, p.431)

Harden (1996) is a great advocate of the approach to education which she describes as 'critical' pedagogy. She detects further problems with andragogy, seeing influences from society as having already been laid prior to individuals entering nurse training, their ideologies about the way in which the world operates already having been formed. She sees a need for the development of nurses as critical individuals who can reappraise social situations rather than simply playing along with them as has previously been the case. Harden also sees the need for counter-oppressive strategies to be adopted by nurses. These ideas may sound extremely laudable and I certainly do agree with the goals. The '*creation*' of nurses who could overcome the oppressive nature of much of the practical detail with which they are confronted is a superb idea. If this sort of nurse could be '*produced*', it would be wonderful. Having said this, it is the very notions which I have just stressed — creation and production — which concern me most. Despite the impressive arguments put forward by many nurse theorists, nurses are still being created and produced from a group of people who knew little about nursing before entering the fray. In other words, they are being influenced — they have to be — by the thoughts of their educators. Of course, this is the only way in which nurses, social workers and teachers can be produced. So the issue of power, the central concept of my current discussion, inevitably comes to the fore. Clare (1993) makes very clear the view that health and educational institutions have enormous power in 'socialising' nurses to be what they want them to be. Students, both before and after qualifying, are required to conform. The reality of the idea of the autonomous, individual nurse who can influence significant change, may still be some distance from us.

There is one further topic which I wish to raise in my discussion of education — the much written about theory-practice gap. The experience of nurses is hugely predominant in practice. Following their training, nurses generally spend little time in educational establishments. Practice nurses, that is those nurses who see the practice of nursing as meaning much more than the 'theory', are highly suspicious and very mistrusting of nursing theory. Those nurses who are attracted to the theoretical side of nursing, generally accept that the practice orientation of most nurses dominates and that what they think or believe about it cannot be utilised. So, here there is another example of power having an impact on the way in which nursing operates. Kelly (1996) undertook a study of graduate nurses and their experience of the first year of registered nursing practice. Some of the findings in this particular study are a little shocking. This group of nurses apparently anticipated fitting in with hospital practice while still retaining their values about nursing. A few problems arose! The nurses felt that power was held by the hospital system and the ward sister or charge nurse. Kelly suggests that senior management has prejudicial attitudes towards graduate nurses. Furthermore, she refers to Cox's (1987) study in which 82 per cent of staff nurses had been subjected to verbal abuse by other nurses. In fact, these clashes as well as conflicts with management, led to the resignation of many nurses. Kelly's study revealed many problems for the graduates she interviewed. The nurses felt that they had problems related to role anxiety. They were concerned about maintaining

> *professional standards despite the lack of resources, inadequate staffing levels on the ward, lack of support, and a sense of responsibility for the standards of others.*
>
> (Kelly, 1996, p.1065)

Other problems are described. The graduate nurses lacked practical experience, they were confronted with unrealistic management expectations and inadequate staffing (which shows up a number of times), were expected to conform, felt that they could not protect patients, and so on. In fact, eight out of the ten nurses interviewed left hospital nursing. A very revealing study. Maybe this is one of the major problems in trying to produce nurses of a high academic standard — that the rest of nursing will be so suspicious of them that they will be rejected, driven out. The theoreticians, the lecturers and the people they teach — in whatever way they teach them — appear to be having little impact at the front line of practice. The problem seems to be a distinct dislike of theoretical nursing amongst nurses who practice and do little else.

Of course, theoreticians have had some impact. One example is the movement in nursing which brought in the 'nursing process' and the current emphasis on holistic practice. Here is a means by which nursing could be viewed as being a distinct professional discipline (Rodgers, 1991), different and distinct from medicine which takes a very objective view of patients and their diseases. To doctors, patients present as an observable set of symptoms to be diagnosed and treated. For nurses today, there is much more to patients. They are people who are ill, for sure, but they are also people who have families, thoughts and feelings, interests, pursuits, and perhaps particular spiritual beliefs as well. In other words, for nurses, patients are much, much more than merely sets of symptoms. For those who deal with the theoretical side of nursing, and also for those who have an interest in pursuing the truly professional interests of nursing — and the many pay-offs which true professionalism brings — this is particularly important. True professions have a separate, distinct body of knowledge from any other occupation, and this is one of the things to be established before true professionalism can be attained. Whilst much of the research and knowledge-chasing may well be in the interests of patients, it may well also be in the 'professional' interests of nurses, from where they will gain more power — at least that is the 'theory'.

I have taken a look at power in an admittedly brief way. Theories about power and how it operates socially are very varied and there are a huge number of them which I have not mentioned here. My aim has been to provide an overview of the various sources from which power emanates to affect nurses and their practice. I have certainly not covered all the areas. There are more — the ethical requirements of the nurse, the law, the Professional Code of Conduct (UKCC, 1992) — all of which force the nurse to act in certain ways in particular situations. The managerial hierarchy and the policies which it produces have a major impact on the way nurses practice. Nurses know that if they do not follow management policy and they make a mistake, it could mean the sack. The difference between the major aims of nurses and their management — cost for managers, care for nurses — is one source of particular conflict. Of course, the origin of this conflict lies in government which year after year sees the cost of care for patients increasing in an era where people live longer. Unfortunately, it is the nurses who pay as the resources available to them decrease. Nurses also feel the influence of the medical profession, telling them what to do, issuing orders which they are expected to follow. The power of the medical profession dominates the health arena and nurses are not in a position to challenge it, despite their numbers. Whilst education might be expected to be a source of comfort to nurses, it too can create problems for them. Many nurses are uncomfortable about nursing theory, feeling much more at ease with the practice routines which have been established over many years and which are difficult for the new diploma or graduate nurse to challenge. It is perhaps not surprising that many nurses are unhappy. They are highly stressed, feel unrewarded, disregarded and underpaid. And these days, more and more are quitting. So, what is the answer? Maybe one step forward would be a serious consideration of how power — or the lack of it — affects the way in which nurses care.

References

Adams T (1991) The idea of revolution in the development of nursing theory. *J Adv Nurs* **16**: 1487–1491

Balsamo D, Martin IS (1995) Developing the sociology of health in nurse education: towards a more critical curriculum — Part 1: andragogy and sociology in Project 2000. *Nurse Educ Today* **15**: 427–432

Brewer AM, Lok P (1995) Managerial strategy and nursing commitment in Australian Hospitals. *J Adv Nurs* **21**: 789–99

Clare J (1993) A challenge to the rhetoric of emancipation: recreating a professional culture. *J Adv Nurs* **18**: 1033–8.
Cox H (1987) in Kelly B (1996) Hospital nursing: 'It's a battle!' A follow-up study of English graduate nurses. *J Adv Nurs* **24**: 1063–9
Cook S (1992) Is professionalism a con? *Nurs Stand* **6** (37): 53–5
Dingwall R, Lewis P, eds (1983) in Sweet SJ, Norman IJ (1995) The nurse-doctor relationship: a selective literature review. *J Adv Nurs* **22**: 165–70
Farmer B (1993) The use and abuse of power in nursing. *Nurs Stand* **7** (23): 33–6
French J, Raven B (1959) in Hewison A (1995) Nurses' power in interactions with patients. *J Adv Nurs* **21**: 75–82
Friedson E (1975) in Hart N (1985) *The Sociology of Health and Medicine.* Causeway Press Ltd, London, UK
Gilbert T (1995) Nursing: empowerment and the problem of power. *J Adv Nurs* **21**: 865–71
Gordon NS, Wimpenny P (1996) A critical reflection on the personal impact of managerial hegemony within nurse education. *J Adv Nurs* **23**: 479–86
Harden J (1996) Enlightenment, empowerment and emancipation: the case for critical pedagogy in nurse education. *Nurse Educ Today* **16**: 32–7
Hewison A (1995) Nurses' power in interactions with patients. *J Adv Nurs* **21**: 75–82
Hokanson Hawks J (1991) Power: a concept analysis. *J Adv Nurs* **16**: 754–62
Illich I (1981) *Medical Nemesis: The Expropriation of Health.* Penguin, London, UK
Jacono B, Jacono J (1994) Power tactics and their potential impact on nursing. *J Adv Nurs* **19**: 954–9
Kelly B (1996) Hospital nursing: 'It's a battle!' A follow-up study of English graduate nurses. *J Adv Nurs* **24**: 1063–9
May C (1995) Patient autonomy and the politics of professional relationships. *J Adv Nurs* **21**: 83–7
Porter S (1992) The poverty of professionalization: a critical analysis of strategies for the occupational advancement of nursing. *J Adv Nurs* **17**: 720–6
Purdy M (1997) Humanist ideology and nurse education. 1. Humanist educational theory. *Nurse Educ Today* **17**: 192–5
Pyne R (1994) Empowerment through the use of the Professional Code of Conduct. *Br J Nurs* **3** (12): 631–4
Rodgers BL (1991) Deconstructing the dogma in nursing knowledge and practice. *Image J Nurs Sch* **23** (3): 177–81
Sweet SJ, Norman IJ (1995) The nurse-doctor relationship: a selective literature review. *J Adv Nurs* **22**: 165–70

Taylor G (1995) Politics and nursing: an elective experience. *J Adv Nurs* **21**: 1180–5
UKCC (1992) *Professional Code of Conduct.* UKCC, London
Wilding P (1982) *Professional Power and Social Welfare.* Routledge & Kegan Paul, London

7

On being silenced: Insights from Foucault and Habermas

Dave Gillespie

Nurses perform a particular role — a particular function — in society. They are the carers, the people who look after those suffering from illness in hospitals, and their role is clearly defined. Nursing history is built upon attitudes of unquestioning obedience; nurses are not the ones to make noises when they are oppressed or feel unhappy with something in which they are involved. They carry out the tasks they are asked, or ordered to do without complaint. Whilst following instructions, which originate from management or medicine for example, they may hide a certain unhappiness, a certain sense of disagreement. However, should they attempt to make their feelings known — for many nurses, a risky strategy — more often than not their concerns are ignored and not taken into account. Nurses who question or disagree are rare and may even be thought of as being quite unusual. Nurses are considered by some poeple to be an oppressed group. With nursing consisting predominantly of women, the subordination and oppression which women experience in life generally is reflected in their role as nurses. They remain silent despite any — or perhaps the many — worries they may have. But why is this? Nurses constitute the largest group of workers within the healthcare system. My understanding is that there are currently around 500,000 nurses working in the UK. Yet their tendency, within the particular groups in which they work in different hospitals, is to put up with all manner of problems at work — stress, lack of resources, poor pay, feelings that they are unimportant, undervalued, and even unvaluable. Still they remain silent. Or have they been silenced? And, if so, how?

There are certain philosophical and sociological theories which may shed some light on how it is that individuals and society in general, and nurses in particular in this case, are controlled; how they are made to conform. One of the most provocative theories is that of Michel Foucault, a post-structuralist French philosopher. Foucault was interested in societal power and how it operated. Whilst his work was unfinished — sadly he died from AIDS in 1984 — the work that he had completed threw a fascinating and perhaps explanatory light on many issues. His theories seem an excellent way of understanding how it is that nurses, amongst others, have been — and often remain — subordinated and oppressed. However, there are some who find Foucault's theory nihilistic, the most vociferous of these probably being Jurgen Habermas whose work is held in high esteem by nurse authors. It is certainly worth considering the thoughts of both these men.

Michel Foucault

Arguably the most provocative thinker of recent times, Foucault's genealogical examinations of (amongst other things) psychiatry, the penal system and sexuality, have provided theoreticians in many different fields with much to consider. The received wisdom of those persuaded by the 'rational' (versus the irrational) has been sharply and directly confronted by Foucault. His works cover a variety of issues and are associated most commonly with subjects such as knowledge and power, discourse, genealogy and archaeology. His focus on the issues of discourse and power has illuminated, in a novel way, the manner in which society has come to be formed, and stands in direct contrast to the previous work of structuralists such as Parsons (1954). Far from seeing society as being structured in a way which is ultimately beneficial to all, Foucault explores the insidious and subjectifying nature of dominant discourses and their power to shape and mould individuals. The notion of the creation of the subject — the 'individual with a mind' (Mautner T, 1997) — in Foucault's work is a fascinating train of thought.

In Foucault's view, 'discipline "makes" individuals' through the means of correct training (Rabinow, 1984, p.188). Throughout his work, Foucault makes apparent the strong relationship between power and knowledge, seeing them both, in fact, as sides of the same coin — the oft-seen power/knowledge formulation. The growth of disciplinary technology is an evolutionary process which is intertwined with the normative social sciences to produce 'the modern individual as a docile and mute body' (Dreyfus and Rabinow, 1986, p.143). The disciplinary exercise of power to produce subjects is based on knowledge — knowledge of persons. Foucault traces the development of institutions — the prison, the hospital, the asylum, the school — through the period since the Middle Ages and regards these institutions as ideal models for the establishment of a pervasive knowledge about persons. Henderson (1994) discusses 'the means of correct training'. Such disciplinary training rests on the idea of 'the gaze', that is, the systematic observation and recording of, for example, physiological pathology and the categorising and collation of these observations. Through this process, the subject of the patient is reduced to the object of medical knowledge (Henderson, 1994). Of course, the hospital provides the ideal environment for this gradual accumulation of knowledge about bodies. According to Foucault, this knowledge forms the basis of institutional power. The ideal institution is based on the army camp:

> *In the perfect camp, all power would be exercised solely through exact observation; each gaze would form a part of the overall functioning of power.*
>
> (Rabinow, 1984, p.189)

Henneman (1995) contends that 'discipline is an important force in maintaining power and limiting and producing knowledge.' In referring to Foucault (1975), the aim of disciplinary technology is of forging a 'docile body that may be subjected, used, transformed, and improved' (Henneman, 1995). Foucault describes the three instruments of discipline: hierarchical observation, normalising judgment and the examination (Rabinow, 1984, pp.189–205).

Hierarchical observation, that is the maintenance of control through surveillance, was established in key institutions. Based on the panoptical — the all-seeing — model of the army camp, 'working-class housing estates, hospitals, asylums, prisons, schools...' were established and soon provided 'the spatial "nesting" of hierarchical surveillance' (Rabinow, 1984, p.190).

Within such institutions, normalising judgment could operate. Michel Foucault, according to Dreyfus and Rabinow (1986, p.158), interestingly describes this judgment as a kind of 'micro-penalty' in which smaller, more trivial areas of life are invidiously accessed and brought under control — areas which fall outside the sweep of the judiciary, for example, lateness, absence, inattention, negligence, insolence, impurity and indecency.

Finally, surveillance and judgment are brought together in the examination. 'In this ritual, the modern form of power and the modern form of knowledge — that of individuals in both cases — are brought together in a single technique' (Dreyfus and Rabinow, 1986, p.158). The examination, in whichever institution it occurs, is for Foucault the focus of power. With the coming of the examination came a transformation of power. Formerly, power had been a highly visible phenomenon, being demonstrated through public manifestations of the force of the sovereign — namely public torture and execution. But now, power was metamorphosed and invisible. Power became shrouded under the veil of beneficence. However, the objects of this power became highly visible — surveyed, judged and examined. The objectifying nature of this process produced what Foucault terms 'docile bodies', normalised individuals, controlled and regulated.

The Foucauldian notion of 'the docile body', bereft of freedom of choice or agency, has drawn criticism from certain quarters, perhaps predominantly from those of the humanist persuasion. Humanistic principles rest on the notions of freedom, choice and agency. Indeed, the humanists were responsible in large part for the 'moral' reform of the asylums and prisons, which had been sharply criticised for their brutality. The new 'moral treatment' of the insane introduced an apparently novel and refreshing approach to helping them. Under the direction of Tuke at the York Retreat in England, and Pinel at the Bicetre and Salpetriere hospitals in France, the shackles and chains of the harsh regimes were removed and replaced with new 'treatments' based on a programme of benevolence and occupational diversion (Weir, 1992).

The philanthropic attitude which underlay these innovations is treated with more than a hint of suspicion by Foucault. He generates an anti-history which attempts to expose the dramatic twist of events which occurred with the advent of moral treatment:

> *The legends of Pinel and Tuke transmit mythical values, which nineteenth century psychiatry would accept as obvious in nature. But beneath the myths themselves, there was an operation, or rather a series of operations, which silently organised the world of the asylum, the methods of cure, and at the same time the concrete experience of madness.*
>
> (Foucault, 1971; p.243)

A close examination of the change in attitudes to and treatment of psychiatric patients, reveals for Foucault a subtle but far-reaching significance. Using the treatment of a young psychiatric patient to illustrate his point, Foucault shows how the introduction to the new regime of comparative liberty, and the removal of old manacles, causes a shift in responsibility. The psychiatric patient is now expected to restrain himself for fear of a return to the old ways.

Hence:

> *there is no question of limiting a liberty that knows no bounds... . The obscure guilt that once linked transgression and unreason is thus shifted; the madman, as a human being once endowed with reason, is no longer guilty of being mad; but the madman, as a madman, and in the interior of that disease of which he is no longer guilty, must feel morally responsible for everything within him that may disturb morality and society, and must hold no one but himself responsible for the punishment that he receives.*
>
> (Foucault, 1971, p.246)

Foucault goes on to state that the:

> *liberation of the insane, abolition of constraint, constitution of a human milieu — these are only justifications... . In fact Tuke created an asylum where he substituted for the free terror of madness the stifling anguish of responsibility; fear no longer reigned on the other side of the prison gates, it now raged under the seals of conscience.*
>
> (Foucault, 1971, p.247)

Thus, the psychiatric patient submits to self-control, to self-discipline. He is now normalised; produced through a process of panoptical surveillance within the asylum walls, and the normalising judgment of his carers. He is returned to 'sanity' — a state decreed by the accepted wisdom of morality and reason.

For Foucault then, in this early example of the normalisation process, notions of freedom are submerged under a gloss of pseudo-liberation. Furthermore, his conflictual relationship with humanism was not bound by the walls of the asylums. His considerations of the control of bodies extended out from the institutional bases of the asylums, prisons and schools to reach out to the wider population.

> *... Disciplines are no longer the prerogative of certain institutions... Disciplines become ubiquitous and liberated... and... are addressed to all people without distinction.*
>
> (Ewald in Armstrong, 1992, pp.169–170)

Foucault envisages a self-disciplining society, '... a judgment of self by self' (Ewald in Armstrong, 1992, p.171) — an individualisation process facilitated by hierarchical surveillance, normalising judgment and the examination. The disciplinary society is now revealed. But what purpose does this society serve? O'Neill (1986) makes a connection between the needs of society with the advent of the industrial age and the correlative need to discipline it. He sees industry and economics as requiring a certain type of individual. In referring to Foucault's (1980) notions of 'anatomopolitics of the body' and 'bio-politics of the population', he highlights the disciplining of bodies as a necessity to the optimisation of production:

> *The articulation of the disciplinary society in the factory, prison, army, schools and hospitals represented a response to social and moral problems arising from industrial change and conflict.*
>
> (O'Neill, 1986)

The seat of power had moved slowly but inexorably from the highly visible mode of the public displays of the feudal era. O'Neill also discusses the role of the state as being:

> *at first minimal in the sense that it served to sweep away the feudal order and to institute the necessary discipline of the new labour force... the state's task in softening domination with education is shared by humanitarian, paternal and religious welfare in helping the poor, the sick, criminal and ignorant.*

He goes on to argue that Foucault (1979) saw the establishment of the disciplinary institutions as:

> *conceived to open up a field for the practices of evaluating, recording and observing large populations in order to administer them through the therapeutic institutions of health, education and penality.*
>
> (O'Neill, 1986)

The irresistible spread of power through a network of disciplinary institutions, touching the lives of all. O'Neill cites Foucault:

> *The moment that saw the transition from historico-ritual mechanisms for the formation of individuality to the scientific-disciplinary mechanism, when the normal took over from the ancestral, and measurement from status, thus substituting for the individuality of the memorable man that of the calculable man, that moment when the sciences of man became possible is the moment when a new technology*

> *of power and a new political anatomy of the body were implemented.*
>
> (Foucault (1980) in O'Neill, 1986)

Foucault, therefore, sees the new sciences, including psychology and sociology — the human sciences — as culpable in the networking of power. Thus, we appear to be presented with a gridlocked situation of all individuals being trapped by the inescapable grip of power. Nobody is self-directing; people are moulded and shaped by the disciplinary society into objects required by the needs of that same society — the modernist society. Of course, this position has attracted many dissenters. The humanists, who are the target of much of Foucault's criticism, react with vigour to Foucault's theory. Perhaps one of their major criticisms of his formulation of power is that Foucault does not provide for an opposite. Patton (1989) refers to Taylor (1984) as thinking that:

> *Foucault's concept of power is incoherent, because he uses the term in a way which does not oppose it to freedom. He wants to discredit as somehow based on a misunderstanding the very idea of liberation from power. But I am arguing that power, in his sense, does not make sense without at least the idea of liberation.*
>
> (Taylor, 1984)

Here, Foucault's position is viewed as lacking an escape from the all-encompassing grasp of power networks. In response to Taylor's criticisms, Patton (1989) proposes an avenue of relief from this apparently impossible position with a re-reading of Foucault's thought. He states that:

> *Foucault is not a philosopher of consciousness concerned to describe or to theorize the experience of attempting to overcome internal limits to freedom. Rather, his concern is with the external supports of the forms of social consciousness and being. He attempts to chart some of the institutions, practices and bodies of knowledge which help to define particular types of individuality.*

This is what Hacking (1986) has described as 'making up people'. However, Patton (1989) also sees that:

> *A range of penal, quasi-penal and therapeutic agencies in modern society practice this sort of identification of people,*

> *imposing identities which serve not only to discriminate between kinds of people, but to fix some in subordinate relations to particular authorities.*

A plausible reference to nurses? For Foucault, individuals are produced by institutions, practices and bodies of knowledge in contrast to the humanist notion that people create themselves through indulging freedom, choice and agency. It would appear that this difference in thought has possibly produced something of a stalemate. Whilst Foucault may help nurses to understand their plight, for them his theories may also be seen as portraying an extremely depressing situation. The position in which they now find themselves may be inescapable. They may be trapped. However, there are other thinkers who offer the possibility of freedom, of emancipation. One such thinker is the German, Jurgen Habermas, who in offering such escape is also one of Foucault's sternest critics.

Jurgen Habermas

Influenced by the Frankfurt School, Habermas has been at the forefront of the philosophical defence of modernism. He has been steadfast in his belief in modernity and defended it from the assault it has endured from authors of the postmodern and poststructuralist era. Critical social theory is perhaps the best known of Habermas' theories and is 'grounded in the critique of dominant ideologies' (Heslop, 1997). White (1995) discusses the emergent criticisms of modernity which arose during the first half of the twentieth century. He highlights in particular works by Heidegger (1946, 1949), and Adorno and Horkheimer (1949) as developing the claim that:

> *enlightened reason and freedom had the ironic long-term effect of engendering new forms of irrationality and repression.*
>
> (White, 1995, p.3)

These critiques had the effect of bringing into question the 'prevailing interpretations of reason, progress, nature, and subjectivity...' (White, 1995, p.3). Horkheimer first coined the term 'critical theory' in the 1930s. It would have:

> *the role of giving new life to the ideals of reason and freedom by revealing their false embodiment in scientism,*

> *capitalism, the 'culture industry', and bourgeois Western political institutions.*
>
> (White, 1995, p.4)

After the second world war, Horkheimer and Adorno re-established the institute at the University of Frankfurt. One of the younger philosophers was called Jurgen Habermas. Unlike Horkheimer and Adorno, who had over time become increasingly disillusioned (Adorno developing a mode of thinking which he called 'negative dialectics' and Horkheimer being drawn to theology), Habermas believed that:

> *one could retain the power of his predecessors' critique of modern life only by clarifying a distinctive conception of rationality and affirming the notion of a just or 'emancipated' society that would somehow correspond to that conception.*
>
> (White, 1995; p.5)

Tensions thus developed between Habermas' thinking and that of 'not only Nietzsche, Heidegger, Foucault, and Derrida, but also Horkheimer and Adorno' (White, 1995, p.5).

Habermas' chosen task was to develop a more comprehensive conception of reason:

> *'... a broader conception that one could begin to sketch the outlines of an 'emancipated' or 'rational' society.*
>
> (White 1995; p.6)

In *Knowledge and Human Interests* (Habermas, 1971), Habermas sets out his thoughts about the existence of:

> *three anthropologically deep-seated interests of human beings, to which three categories of knowledge and rationality correspond. We have 'knowledge-constitutive' interests in the* [a] *technical control of the world around us, in* [b] *understanding others, and in* [c] *freeing ourselves from structures of domination: a 'technical', a 'practical', and an 'emancipatory' interest.*
>
> (White 1995, p.6)

In man's pursuit of the technical domination of nature, he has engendered a technical domination over human beings. The correction of this unbalanced distortion lies in what Habermas considers to be a necessary reaffirming of 'the rationality inherent in our "practical" and "emancipatory" interests' (White, 1995, p.6). This emancipatory interest is modelled on psychoanalysis and is:

> *rooted in our ability to act and think self-consciously, to reason and make decisions on the basis of facts known about a situation and the socially accepted rules that govern interaction.*
>
> (Craib, 1984, p.206)

Habermas points to distortions in communication and decision-making processes, for example, where one party is unaware of all the facts or where rules prevent their full and complete participation. It is critical science's role to correct these distortions and to lead to true emancipation.

Habermas' project took a certain turn with his 'exploration of the on-going "communicative competence" displayed by all speakers of natural languages' (Habermas in White, 1995, pp. 6–7). This spawned his work on, 'the theory of communicative action'. At the centre of human reason, according to Habermas, lies this communicative activity. There exists a fundamental link between communicative action and rationality:

> *... the theory of communicative action and rationality generates more conceptual, moral, and empirical insight than alternative approaches.*
>
> (Habermas, in White, 1995, p.7)

One important context for this is highlighted as being methodological discussions in the social sciences. In addition, White (1995, p.7) refers to Habermas as encouraging interconnectedness between academic disciplines and their studies.

The theory of communicative action is best known for the striking perspective it provides on how we should understand modernity, the period during which such concepts as democracy, capitalism, belief in science, and commitment to humanitarian principles were established.

> *Habermas offers a two-level interpretation of the modern world, in which a distinction is drawn between the rational potential implicit in 'cultural modernity' and the selective or one-sided utilization of that potential in 'societal processes of modernization'.*
>
> (White, 1995; p.8)

Habermas discusses the notion of the 'rationalized lifeworld' where:

> *actors consistently carry the expectation that the various validity claims raised in speech are to be cognitively distinguished, and that they have to be redeemed in different ways. As such a lifeworld emerges, an increasing number of spheres of social interaction are removed from guidance by unquestioned tradition and opened to co-ordination through consciously achieved agreement.*
>
> (White, 1995, p.8)

Simultaneously, 'there also occurs an advance in the rationality of society... '. This latter sort of rationalisation means that there is an expansion of social subsystems which coordinate action through the media of money (capitalist economy) and administrative power (modern, centralized states). The initially beneficial expansion of these media has progressed to the point, however, where they increasingly invade areas of social life which have been, or could be, coordinated by the medium of understanding or 'solidarity'. Modernisation in the West has thus generated a pathology: an unbalanced development of its potential.

> *Habermas sees palpable signs of the rejection of the smooth unfolding of functionalist reason in various new social movements that have emerged since the 1960s... . Whether the questions arise in the form of a critique of productivist civilization as in the ecological movement, or in the form of a rejection of scripted identities as in feminism or the gay and lesbian rights movement, they all constitute resistance points to further colonization*
>
> (White, 1995, pp.8–9)

Habermas is not without his critics. His universalism — the belief that all human beings are equal (Mautner, 1997), has produced broadsides from poststructuralist, postmodern, and feminist thinkers alike. They see this universalism as functioning merely:

> *to blind the West to the ways in which it both drives itself in ever more disciplinary directions and engenders 'others' who fall short of the demands carried by its criteria of reason and responsibility.*
>
> (White, 1995, p.9).

For Habermas, Foucault's theories:

> *lack a mechanism for social integration such as language, with its interlacing of performative attitudes of speakers and hearers, which could explain the individuating effects of socialization… . Foucault compensates for this by purifying the concept of individuation of all connotations of self-determination and self-realization, and reducing it to an inner world produced by external stimuli and fitted out with arbitrarily manipulable, representative contents.*
>
> (Kelly, 1994; p.99)

The issue here, states Habermas:

> *is whether the model of an inflation of the psychic that is evoked by power techniques (or released by the disintegration of the institutions) does not make it necessary to bring the growth in subjective freedom under descriptions that render unrecognizable the experience of an expanded scope for expressive self-manifestation and for autonomy.*
>
> (Habermas in Kelly, 1994, p.99)

Habermas goes on to further criticise Foucault's general thoughts about the transformations of disciplinary power he has indicated, for example the veneer of humanism (or humanitarianism) which shrouded the reform of the penal system:

> *Foucault wants to show that beneath this was concealed a brutal change in the practices of power — the modern regime of power... the thesis is false in its generality.*
>
> (Habermas in Kelly, 1994, p.100)

Habermas highlights a number of deficiencies, which move gradually through the development of the moral-ethical positions of deontology and utilitarianism, and which concentrate on the issues of language and 'internal aspects of the development of law' (Habermas in Kelly, 1994, p.101), to culminate in his final and perhaps most critical response to Foucault, regarding his neglect of:

> *the development of normative structures in connection with the modern formation of power. As soon as Foucault takes up the threads of the biopolitical establishment of disciplinary power, he lets drop the threads of the legal organization of the exercise of power and of the legitimation of the order of domination… . As soon as he*

passes from the classical to the modern age, Foucault pays no attention whatsoever to penal law and to the law governing the penal process.

(Habermas in Kelly, 1994, pp.101–102)

What Habermas appears to be indicating here is an endorsement of the reform of the penal system brought about by the development of a more humanitarian approach. It could be suggested, by extension, that Habermas allies himself to humanism and to the Enlightenment project — basically man's development of reasoned thinking, in sharp contrast to Foucault's critique of these very things. In very simple terms, the reform of prisons has not, as in Foucault's view, furthered the brutality of the system, but ameliorated a great deal of its excesses.

Foucault died in 1984 and is, therefore, unable to provide replies to the many criticisms focused on him by, amongst others, Habermas. One question perhaps needs to be asked: Is nursing (and, therefore, are individual nurses) merely a product of a disciplinary system, or are nurses autonomous to the extent that they have overcome the apparent distortions in the communicative system? Are they trapped, are they free, or are they somewhere in between?

Foucault, viewed by most writers as belonging to the post-structuralist school, has come in for both support and criticism from many nursing authors. Mulholland (1995) refers to Foucault and his disenchantment with humanism. The transmitted humanist beliefs suggest that human beings have the ability to transcend power. This particular belief is a fundamental aspect of humanism and places the rational human being in a position of dominance. As Mulholland states, 'the capacity for reason distinguishes humanity from nature and facilitates its capacity for freedom' (Mulholland 1995, p.444). This position places the human subject at the ontological — the theory of being — centre of human history. This is the belief which has been adopted by nursing culture: that nurses are capable of creating and are free to create themselves. The freedom and liberation with which nurses operate is inevitably transmitted further on to the patients for whom they care. However, Mulholland is not entirely convinced by this representation of humanism and refers to Foucault (1977):

The notion of a constituent subject is a humanist mystification that occludes a critical examination of the various

> *institutional sites where subjects are produced within power relations.*

This is obviously a very different position from that of the humanists. Far from people having the freedom to create themselves they are, in fact, produced via power relations within institutional arenas. Here Mulholland has brought to his readers' attention the possible problems with humanistic theory.

The key issue which is emerging is that nurses (and other healthcare professionals) are far from 'free' and able to be 'self-creative'. Their work is largely influenced and constrained by policies. These policies, whether local or national, may have been developed 'elsewhere' and by 'outsiders' and imposed upon healthcare staff. So we cannot separate actions from policies, power and issues of control.

Here, again, is the suggestion that the 'free' nurse suggested by humanistic theory is being controlled and dominated by institutional power. Indeed, the pervasive role of power is seen by some authors as being more widespread than merely the particular institution where the nurse works. The educational system, which these days plays a large part in the functioning of nursing staff, is seen as possessing a particularly powerful influence. Dispenza (1996), whilst referring to many other authors, includes Foucault's thought by recognising that the desire for relationships of equality between lecturers and students is undermined by the notion that lecturers have greater knowledge and, therefore, greater power than students. Henneman (1995) refers to Foucault in great depth in her attempt to throw light upon the apparent lack of collaboration between doctors and nurses and the disproportionate share of power between them.

Whilst these authors have found ways in which Foucault's thought can be utilised to understand and appreciate certain issues related to nursing practice and education, there are other authors who are sceptical about Foucault's thesis and postmodernism and poststructuralism in general. Kermode and Brown (1996) argue strongly against the postmodern movement, of which Foucault is described as a member. They refer to Sarup (1988) who suggests that:

> *postmodernists... offer no theoretical reason to move in any particular social direction. In this respect, post-modernism is not an agent of social change but an agent of social stasis.*
>
> (Kermode and Brown, 1996, p.379)

This is perhaps the most common criticism of postmodernism — the idea that it offers no way out; that it only offers the alternative of entrapment. As Porter (1996) states:

> *the danger of accepting Foucault's conception of power too readily is that, despite its apparent radicalism, it leads to praxical paralysis.*
>
> (Porter, 1996, p.76)

Kermode and Brown (1996) also refer to Hartsock (1990) who argues that:

> *postmodernism only manages to criticise the theories of European modernism without putting anything in their place... Foucault and others... 'fail'... to provide an epistemology which is capable of revolutionising, creating, and constructing.*
>
> (Kermode and Brown, 1996, p.379)

On the other hand, the nursing literature (which I have read) has nothing but appreciation (apparently) for the Habermasian approach. There are numerous papers which demonstrate the practical usage of critical social theory. Wells (1995) performs a thorough appraisal of this theory in her description of critical theory and its use, for example, in the discharge decision-making process. She points out:

> *as Habermas' theory indicates, communicative action does not arise, because it is colonized or displaced by a strategic orientation, which also allows professionals to control the process.*
>
> (Wells, 1995, p.54)

Wells highlights the lack of communicative action as being a fundamental missing link in this procedure. Wilson-Thomas (1995) sees critical social theory as a liberatory device. She says this process '... aims to analyse the constraints of the cultural context and replace them with emancipatory ideologies' (Wilson-Thomas, 1995, p.572). Holmes and Warelow (1997) utilise critical theory to examine the possibility of creating a quite new understanding of human need, suggesting that today's understanding has been hegemonically created and is untrue. They seek to find emancipation from today's understanding through a process of critical reflection bringing about praxis. These are just a few papers — far from all the many which exist — which demonstrate a thorough interest in Habermas' theories by nurse theoreticians. I have found it difficult to locate books or papers which are anti-Habermasian in the nursing field. I may need to apologise for my ignorance. However, in contrast, Kelly (1994) gives a considered defence of Foucault's thinking against the major attacks it has suffered at the hands of Habermas.

Whilst many nurses (myself included) may be attracted to Foucault's explanations of power and how it operates in society, there may well be those who are somewhat dispirited by its apparent failure to offer a way out. Having said this, it is certainly a theory which is worthy of consideration by those working in a highly institutionalised field of work, such as healthcare. It is of great importance for us to understand and comprehend the forces which are at play in maintaining our conformity and our silence. Habermas also offers us a theory by which we may gain some insight into and understanding of the manner in which society has developed and robbed us of our freedom. There exist distinct differences in the two men's thinking, although attention has been drawn to the apparent similarities which have not been presented here. In the light of such theories, our entrapment becomes somewhat easier to see and understand. Having understood our imprisonment, there remains a need to find an escape route and certainly Habermas does give us one potential means of achieving this (a deeper reading of Foucault's work provides another). It must certainly be that nurses would hope that the emancipation from the 'prisons' which some of them currently occupy, is a goal that is achievable.

References

Adorno TW, Horkheimer M (1949) in White SK (1995) *The Cambridge Companion to Habermas.* Cambridge University Press, Cambridge

Craib I (1984) *Modern Social Theory: From Parsons to Habermas.* The Harvester Press Ltd, Brighton

Dispenza V (1996) Empowering students: a pragmatic philosophical approach to management education. *Management Learning* **27** (2): 239–51

Dreyfus HL, Rabinow P (1986) *Michel Foucault: Beyond Structuralism and Hermeneutics.* The Harvester Press Ltd, Brighton

Ewald F in Armstrong TJ, ed (1992) *Michel Foucault Philosopher: Essays Translated from the French and German.* Harvester Wheatsheaf, London

Foucault M (1979) in O'Neill J (1986) The disciplinary society: from Weber to Foucault. *Br J Sociol* **37**: 42–60

Foucault M (1980) in O'Neill J (1986) The disciplinary society: from Weber to Foucault. *Br J Sociol* **37**: 42–60

Foucault M (1971) *Madness and Civilisation: a History of Insanity in the Age of Reason.* Tavistock Publications, London.

Foucault M (1975) in Henneman EA (1995) Nurse-physician collaboration: a poststructuralist view. *J Adv Nurs* **22**: 359–63

Foucault M (1977) in Mulholland J (1995) Nursing, humanism and transcultural theory: the 'bracketing-out' of reality. *J Adv Nurs* **22**: 442–9

Habermas J (1971) *Knowledge and Human Interests.* Beacon Press, Boston

Hacking I (1986) in Patton P (1989) Taylor and Foucault on power and freedom. *Political Studies* **37**: 260–76

Hartsock N (1990) in Kermode S, Brown C (1996) The postmodernist hoax and its effects on nursing. *Int J Nurs Stud* **33** (4): 375–84

Heidegger M (1946) in White SK (1995) *The Cambridge Companion to Habermas.* Cambridge University Press, Cambridge

Heidegger M (1949) in White SK (1995) *The Cambridge Companion to Habermas.* Cambridge University Press, Cambridge

Henderson A (1994) Power and knowledge in nursing practice: the contribution of Foucault. *J Adv Nurs* **20**: 935–9

Henneman EA (1995) Nurse-physician collaboration: a poststructuralist view. *J Adv Nurs* **22**: 359–63

Heslop L (1997) The (im)possibilities of poststructuralist and critical social nursing inquiry. *Nurs Inquiry* **4**: 48–56

Holmes CA, Warelow PJ (1997) Culture, needs and nursing: a critical theory approach. *J Adv Nurs* **25**: 463–70

Kelly M (1994) *Critique and Power: Recasting the Foucault/Habermas Debate.* The MIT Press, Cambridge

Kermode S, Brown C (1996) The postmodernist hoax and its effects on nursing. *Int J Nurs Stud* **33** (4): 375–84

Mautner T (1997) *Dictionary of Philosophy.* Penguin Books, London

Mulholland J (1995) Nursing, humanism and transcultural theory: the 'bracketing-out' of reality. *J Adv Nurs* **22**: 442–9

O'Neill J (1986) The disciplinary society: from Weber to Foucault. *Br J Sociol* **37**: 42–60

Parsons T (1954) *Essays in Sociological Theory. The Free Press of Glencoe.* Collier-MacMillan Ltd, London

Patton P (1989) Taylor and Foucault on power and freedom. *Political Stud* **37**: 260–76

Porter S (1996) Contra-Foucault: soldiers, nurses and power. *Sociol* **30** (1): 59–78

Rabinow P (1984) *The Foucault Reader.* Penguin, London

Sarup M(1988) in Kermode S, Brown C (1996) The postmodernist hoax and its effects on nursing. *Int J Nurs Stud* **33** (4): 375–84

Taylor C (1984) in Patton P (1989) Taylor and Foucault on power and freedom. *Political Stud* **37**: 260–76

Weir R (1992) An experimental course of lectures on moral treatment for mentally ill people. *J Adv Nurs* **17**: 390–5

Wells DL (1995) The importance of critical theory to nursing: a description using research concerning discharge decision making. *Can J Nurs Res* **27** (2): 45–58

White SK (1995) *The Cambridge Companion to Habermas.* Cambridge University Press, Cambridge

Wilson-Thomas L (1995) Applying critical social theory in nursing education to bridge the gap between theory, research and practice. *J Adv Nurs* **21**: 568–75

Index

K

L

M

N

O

P

Q

R

S